PRAISE FOR TAKING CONTROL

"This book is beautiful and truly touched my heart to the core. What a brilliant book, so honest, raw, and needed. Taking Control is excellent, and many Muslims could learn a lot from it on the topic of living with infertility."

—Dr Amal Alahmad
Obstetrics, Gynecology and Infertility Consultant

"Wow! What a read. I cried, I nodded, I smiled. I went through the spectrum of emotions and it touched me to the core. I love the author's raw and frank style. I love her positivity. I love the emotional support offered as well as the practical considerations. She's not shy to discuss all the options, which is fantastic."
—Dr Abia Afsar-Siddiqui

"I loved this book so much. Farah is brave to write this book and share her story. There are no books like this on the market and it is sorely needed. The author encourages the reader to find the joy in life despite the hardship of struggling to have a child, as well as practical information on treatments such as IVF and dealing with social pressures. I hope this book is translated into Arabic soon so I can share it with many patients who I work with and who mostly speak Arabic. This book will enlighten the difficulty of TTC as a Muslim woman for many women."

—Adwaa Khudhari, MD
Consultant
Obstetrics & Gynecology
Reproductive Endocrinology & Infertility

TAKING CONTROL

A Muslim Woman's Guide to Surviving Infertility

Farah Dualeh

TUGHRA
BOOKS

ISBN: 978-1-59784-949-4
Ebook: 978-1-59784-983-8

Library of Congress Cataloging-in-Publication Data

Names: Dualeh, Farah, author.
Title: Taking control : a Muslim woman's guide to infertility / Farah
  Dualeh.
Description: New Jersey : Tughra Books, [2022]
Identifiers: LCCN 2022000573 (print) | LCCN 2022000574 (ebook) | ISBN
  9781597849494 (paperback) | ISBN 9781597849838 (ebook)
Subjects: LCSH: Infertility--Religious aspects. | Muslim
  women--Psychological aspects.
Classification: LCC RC889 .D79 2022 (print) | LCC RC889 (ebook) | DDC
  618.1/780088297--dc23/eng/20220125
LC record available at https://lccn.loc.gov/2022000573
LC ebook record available at https://lccn.loc.gov/2022000574

Contents

Acknowledgements 7

Introduction 9

Part 1 TRYING TO CONCEIVE 15

1. My Story and My Approach 17
2. Womanhood and Identity 33
3. The Body and the Period 38
4. In the Company of Greats & Delayed Parenthood 41
5. The Most Difficult Question 45
6. Emotional Support 51
7. Dealing With Social Pressures 61
8. An Awesome Marriage 67
9. What Friends and Family Need to Know - Your Message 77
10. Stories of the Brave 84

Part 2 TREATMENT OPTIONS 97

Part 3 YOUR FAMILY, YOUR OPTIONS 129

Epilogue 149

Endnote 151

I dedicate this book to every Muslim sister struggling to conceive. I also dedicate it, to Allah S.W.T, in the hope that He accepts this small effort and make my scales of good deeds heavier with it. Ameen.

ACKNOWLEDGEMENTS

The process of writing this book was made surprisingly easy for me by the grace of God. I sincerely acknowledge and thank those that have helped make it reality. Thank you to my coach Na'ima B Robert, whose IG post allowed me to take the action to start this book. A massive thank you to Hend Hegazi who helped me edit and make sense of my ideas at the very beginning. Thank you to Umm Suhaila, who was the first person to read the initial draft of this book and supported me all the way through – I appreciate you. Thank you to the amazing people who bravely and generously shared their stories with me – and now you – in chapter 10. A huge thank you to the editor and team at Tughra Books for believing in this message and allowing me to be part of the process to the end. Finally, I thank you Zakaria, my husband, the most generous and loving person I know. I am grateful to experience life with you.

INTRODUCTION

To my dear sister who has been trying to conceive,

My hope is that you have found this book at the moment you started to feel even slightly concerned or confused about your fertility. This is the book I needed from the start of trying to conceive (TTC) and it has been the book I have continued to need ever since. I have written this book so that you will have that support. You will have a place where you can find answers, reassurances and know that you are not alone. That the private worries and thoughts you have are shared with so many amazing women around the world. You are unique and your specific situation will be unique, but I want you to know that there are women like yourself who share your beautiful faith and who also find themselves on the road of navigating through infertility.

I initially felt it was pointless for someone who has been trying to conceive for a shorter period—such as 6 months to a year—to delve into the amount of information presented in this book. I also felt it was unnecessary for them to go to places that this book will take you emotionally; a couple trying to conceive for a year or less are likely to conceive naturally sooner rather than later and therefore this book would be unsuitable for them. However, half-way through writing this book, I changed my mind.

I realised that the book is for all Muslim women or couples TTC right from the beginning of their journey. The time-period of 'starting for TTC' will vary from couple to couple. For some, the concern about their fertility will come to the forefront of their thoughts immediately after trying, and for others it will be much later.

The reason I hope that you have found this book as early in your journey as possible is that the way you start this experience has a lot of influence on how you thrive through it, regardless of how long it lasts.

What you will read in the following pages will affect the questions you need to ask yourself, the mindset you need to adopt, and the coping mechanisms you will want to use. All this is vital to take place as early as possible on the journey so that you can build on those plans and beliefs. It also reduces the length of time you suffer in silence, the length of time you feel confused without anyone to turn to for guidance on this situation.

A situation, I am almost sure, you are unlikely to have considered before marriage or before trying to conceive. Unless you are among the small percentage of women who discover their fertility complications earlier due to a previously established health concern, it likely came as an overwhelming shock.

My wish is that you have found this book early on so you may gain the most benefit from it, but even if you are 4, 9, 15 years into the journey, this resource is still for you. It has been written with you in mind, to provide you with a safe space. This space is yours and it is designed to elevate you. Elevate your perspective and approach to the TTC experience. Elevate your self-love and sense of strong identity despite the test that you face individually and as a couple.

This book was written directly and honestly for you and is constructed to challenge you. It will challenge your outlook and thinking and ask you to reclaim your power on this journey. It asks you to centre yourself on this unpleasant road. It asks you to treat yourself sensitively and with compassion. It asks you to have a sense of agency in your life, to take control, to be proactive, to challenge the status quo, to push back against societal pressures, and to live a life of your choosing as much as possible despite you not choosing to experience infertility.

It asks you to find the balance in being aware and accepting of your feelings whilst avoiding victimhood at all costs. It asks you to know with certainty that happiness on this journey and beyond is possible. And finally, it asks you for confidence that your Creator has your back. He always has and He always will.

This reminder of trusting in Allah/God (true *tawakkul*) is the key reason why this book is not for all women. Women regardless of their country of residence, faith, ethnicity, or age have so much in common on their TTC journey. There is a strange and wonderful sisterhood that is built on understanding each other's pain and experience on this mission and therefore so much that is discussed in this book is relevant and beneficial for many women from all backgrounds and faiths. But please be aware that the language used in this book—which relies heavily on the concept of *tawakkul*—is directed towards Muslim women.

I want to be clear that although this idea of trusting Allah as well the inclusion of Islamic rulings for some of the medical treatments available for infertility is faith-based, this is not an Islamic book. This is not a book that is designed to teach you about Islam nor to provide detailed *fatwas* on any subject.

It is valuable for us to start with the reminder that Islam is perfect and therefore sufficient as a guide in all areas of life as promised by Allah himself: '*This day have I perfected your religion for you, completed My favour upon you, and have chosen for you Islam as your religion*' (Quran 5.3). Therefore, continuously turning back to Allah is the sincerest action we can advise and remind each other, regardless of the situation. However, we are human and as such, we fall short of our religious obligations and sometimes our faith fluctuates.

The result is at times we will find ourselves feeling lost, without direction and our trust in Allah wavering (even though our belief stays intact). In addition to reminders about strengthening our trust in Allah, we also require practical guidelines relevant to this difficulty. For this reason, this book is designed to be a practical guide for you to use as you traverse through this unknown path. It is an aid for you to survive in what often feels like a mum's world, to be used as a tool to gain strength through infertility.

You'll find in this book practical information including chapters on having 'An Awesome Marriage' throughout TTC or dealing with social pressures such as pregnancy announcements and baby showers. You'll also find guidance on treatment options to consider for yourself and your situation.

The best way to utilise this book is to interact with it at every stage by making the content personal to your unique situation. Much of the information is directed at you as if we were face-to-face, and therefore you will reap the most value from it by being actively engaged with the material as a practical guide; a guide to change or improve the uphill battle of surviving infertility. One way to do this is by completing the questions at the end of certain chapters or sections. You can use a journal or a private notebook to work through these important questions.

This book is divided into three separate parts, each covering a different stage or need for the Muslim woman or couple facing infertility. Part 1 is about Navigating the TTC Journey, Part 2 discusses Treatment Options, and Part 3 introduces you to some other Family Options. I encourage you to complete Part 1 before you move on to Parts 2 and 3 as this section deals with mindset as well as strengthening your relationship with your spouse, all of which are necessary to strengthen yourself and your marriage before you can consider any options.

Be sure to engage and complete the questions provided at the end of each section, as this will help you achieve an enhanced level of clarity about your feelings and options whilst trying to conceive. This can help you and your spouse, where appropriate, to formulate an action plan to execute immediately in most cases, or to return to at a later stage. Books can be an incredible vehicle for change and growth, but this can only happen in a measurable way when we put what we learn into practise.

Specific parts of the book are designed to be returned to again and again, revisited as often as you need. The pages of *dua* and reminders are one example of this. Feel free to bookmark and return to any section of the book when the time is right, or you reach that stage of the TTC journey. My prayer is this:

May this book give you solace in the pain of pursuing mother-

hood. May it be a source of light in the darkest of moments. May it give you clarity on what is available and what is possible in starting a family and finding joy in your life. May it change your perspective and heart in a way that serves you, your family, and society at large. May you be even stronger for the experience of reading this book and most importantly putting it into practise. Everything you need is within you and although it will not be an easy battle, this is a battle you can win today by the mindset you choose to adopt. Perspective is everything and you can reframe your experience any time so that it serves you better.

With love
Farah Dualeh

Infertility and Its Causes

Infertility is when a couple cannot get pregnant (conceive) despite having regular unprotected sex. (NHS, 2020). This book won't focus heavily on the causes of infertility but there are several causes of infertility affecting both men and women. Furthermore, in the UK, unexplained infertility accounts for around 1 in 4 cases of infertility. In the US, test results of 5-10% of couples trying to conceive are normal showing no apparent cause for infertility. (American Society of Reproductive Medicine). No matter what's causing your infertility, this book will help you find strength in your journey.

PART 1

TRYING TO CONCEIVE

CHAPTER 1

MY STORY AND MY APPROACH

B orn in a war-torn country. Lost mother in childhood. Left home at 17. Married at 24. And so far, married 12 years with no children.

What a bleak set of unfortunate circumstances, eh? This is a snapshot of some major events in my life that I share with you at this stage, in the hope that it helps you understand my story better on this journey we are about to embark on together.

Just like you, I have had many stages and facets to my life which all make up who I am. The bulk of this chapter will be sharing with you my own experiences of fertility issues and how I have managed to achieve happiness and contentment through an incredibly challenging and unexpected part of my life.

I aim to share this with you, to firstly remind you that you are most definitely not alone on this journey (even though I know it can feel like it) and secondly, to provide a different approach to dealing with infertility in the hope that you can also find happiness and the ability to be content on the path to motherhood.

We will return to my experience with infertility, which is the focus of this chapter, but let me first share with you where it began—where I began—before we examine where I currently am.

I was born in Somalia (East Africa). I was happy being with my family and having simple pleasures, but still, my earliest and key memories from this period are marred by extreme and difficult experiences.

Here are two unforgettable experiences from that period. The first of these memories is during the height of the civil war, when my family and I were escaping with neighbours to safety. En route, we saw many children without adults to care for them.

This left me with the realisation, at a tender age of 6 or 7, that loss and fear are part of life and are often caused by circumstances and situations outside of our control.

The second memory from that period is one of regret, for choices that were seemingly simple at the time. This was missing out on being with my mother in her dying hours and missing out on saying goodbye. You see, my mother was being looked after by my sister in the city whilst the rest of my family remained living as nomads. My mother, sensing her time was close, had requested her youngest child (myself) to stay with her during her last days.

Unfortunately, I used to struggle being in a new environment. My mother seemed to be always sleeping, I was savaged by city mosquitoes, and I missed the rest of my family, especially my dear dad. One day my sister went to her neighbour—or maybe it was to the local shops—and asked me to sit with my mother for a short time. Instead of doing what I was told, I decided to run away. To run back, more precisely, to my dad and to the fresh air I knew so well without mosquitoes.

Let me just say I gave the family an eventful evening full of worry and then startled them further when I arrived unscathed and unharmed to where the rest of the family were. I was impressed with my achievement of finding my way home but any excitement I had over this was short-lived when shortly after I was informed that my mother had passed.

If only I knew how much it would mean to me in later years should I have stayed with her till the end and say goodbye. However, death and loss were not things I was able to comprehend fully at this delicate age.

Within a year of my mum passing, I found myself in a small, cold town in the north of England with only my teenage brother from my immediate family and one of the few people I knew from my old life. But as only children know how, I adapted and found comfort in my new way of life before long. I lived in this town for almost 10 years and then left home at the sweet age of 17 and moved to London.

One of the consequences of my childhood was the deep desire to create and be surrounded by my own nuclear family. The events that formed my childhood—experiencing war, losing my mum and moving away from my nuclear family—were out of my control, but as a young adult, I had the naïve belief that I could control major aspects of my life, aspects like forming a family.

At 24 years old I got married to a lovely man, and after about a year enjoying marriage, we made the conscious decision to start a family. I was excited and took this decision very seriously. The first step I took to prepare for parenthood was researching local parenting courses I could join. I knew being a mum was not something I wanted to do half-heartedly and so we began to try.

By month three of not being pregnant, I was in disbelief. What happened to the endless amounts of information we had been fed in school that just one incident of unprotected sex would result in pregnancy?

Within six months of trying for a baby, my time became consumed by online research on the topic. It was there that I was first introduced to terms such as 'infertility' and 'trying to conceive'. There were hundreds of women on these online forums supporting and consoling each other about their fertility concerns. I was astounded to learn about this issue of infertility and was amazed by how common it turned out to be. I may have had some previous exposure to the topic in real life or through the media, but it was not something that had entered my consciousness or that I considered as a possibility in my own life.

At first, the online support groups provided me with some relief from the confusion. Naively, I also felt that there would be support here to help me understand and overcome what I was experiencing. But the unexpected truth for me was that these spaces had me feeling like an outcast, not fully able to participate in the good-hearted education sharing that was taking place between the want-to-be mums in these groups.

'Why me?' – a common question found in most posts within these forums. Women felt angry and confused as to the 'reason' they were going through this hardship. Some vented and wrote 'how they had been 'good', not smoked, etc. Others talked about 'being ready' and settled in their lives and hence 'motherhood' was their right at this stage in their life. Their pain and frustration were palpable and understandable, but it was incompatible with my beliefs about myself, the world, and my Lord. I found myself unable to relate and thus receive or provide any solace in the support that was available through these platforms. Other common conversations centred around fertility treatment options and personal updates. There was much discussion on IVF/IUI, egg and sperm donors as well as surrogacy. All of it was overwhelming and considerable amounts of it inappropriate for me as a Muslim woman, and for us as a Muslim couple.

During this time and rather unassumingly, it dawned on me that my husband and I were in fact 'struggling to conceive'. It also dawned on me that there was extraordinarily little assistance online or in real life for Muslim women or couples struggling with this health issue. Nevertheless, looking back to that time, I am almost overcome with emotion because whilst I was fearful and highly confused by this unexpected reality, a calmness enveloped me, and I knew that things were going to be ok.

Surprisingly, the more I started to think about the trial of struggling to have a child or potentially being barren, I was filled with hope and curiosity and intrigued by what my Lord may have in store for me.

Next came what I describe as a light during a potentially dark time. This light is ultimately how I have thrived in my life and how my husband and I have thrived as a couple over the past 12 years. What is this light I refer to? It is the 'light' of intentionality. I became extremely intentional about my response to this hardship. My decision became one of taking control. A resolution that my emotions would not 'get away from me', that my emotions, the unfolding of my life, the things I would do or see were not just going to happen to me. Instead, I would be in control. The well-known idea that what defines you is not your circumstance but rather your *response* to the circumstance rang immensely true for me.

There is an idea discussed by Steven R. Covey, in his book; *The Seven Habits of Highly Effective People.* The idea encourages one to be proactive and to focus on what you can control, your 'areas of influence' in life, and the experiences you face. Although I had not yet read this remarkable book, this was exactly what I did and what I continue to do regarding my fertility struggles and for all other areas of life. It truly has been a light for me.

At this point, you might be thinking that this all sounds impossible, an alien concept. You may argue that you are unable to control your emotions, unable to control the heart-breaking disappointments, sadness, and possible depression due to this health problem. Your feelings and thoughts are appropriate. Of course, they are, but I implore you to allow yourself to think differently. I assure you it is possible to take control of your perspective and mindset, and therefore your actions and emotions. It is possible to decide your approach going forward on the challenging path to motherhood. This does not mean you ignore or vilify your sadness or worry about struggling to be a parent; taking control means you choose a way that will give you peace, contentment, and joy along your journey. If you must go on this TTC battle, for however long it may be, you might as well pursue happiness and some light through it; otherwise what is the alternative?

I want you to know that despite being intentional, despite the choice to be happy through this ordeal, I, too, face dark days filled with sadness, worry, confusion, isolation, and embarrassment. I, too, live a life where even during moments of pure joy or achievement, I still feel that something is missing. I, too, have had the names of my children picked out for the longest time and every time a couple (especially newlyweds) name their child the same name, my heart breaks a little in the remembrance of what I am missing.

I'm intimately familiar with the unusual reality of dealing with grief for the 'loss' of the child that never was. I know this sense of loss will be even deeper for those who have experienced a miscarriage whilst being challenged with conceiving. I vividly remember how overcome I was with grief in the early days, the first couple of years of TTC. I was surprised to feel so much love for a child that never was, to feel the presence and then the vanishing for a child that had not yet been conceived. Therefore, know that your feelings, those described on these pages as well those that might be missed in this book altogether, are all valid, just, and understandable. I must reiterate that by encouraging you to choose joy, to find the light, to adopt a perspective that will aid happiness and a sense of moving forward doesn't mean that you do not from time to time feel the harsh reality that is infertility.

In the early days, the shock was the worst. How did I not know about this common problem faced by 1 in 7 couples? This was not the plan. This is not how I had envisioned a married life. I am a planner and I try to control. This is me in my approach to many aspects of life. I feel that this characteristic of mine made the early days noticeably harder, but I was humbled by the words of Allah when He said 'they plan, and Allah plans. Surely Allah is the best of planners' (Quran 8:30).

As a result of my initial obsessive google research into this new world I found myself in, I came across expert recommendations that advised couples trying for a baby to see their General Practitioner (GP) (Primary Care Physician – PCP – in the US) in specified time frames. It stated that couples where the woman is aged below 35, to see their GP after naturally trying to conceive for up to 12 months. For those aged over 35, 6 months was the recommendation.

My husband and I promptly went to our doctor and were reassured that things should all be fine but would be referred for further tests. We went on to have many tests. I say "we," but I mean "me," because, let's face it, for the male partner the initial phase during most fertility testing or treatments is a simple semen analysis to determine sperm health on mobility and volume, whereas the female is tested and prodded extensively. Below are several tests or methods I had in the initial phase:

* Virology test
* Day two hormone profile
* AMH level
* 3D scan and antral follicle count
* FSH
* Ovarian Reserve check
* Laparoscopy
* Blood test for all hormones

As my results were always normal or average, we were reassured at each point of the testing phase that we were extremely likely to fall naturally pregnant whilst we continued with routine tests. From the results of our tests and their years of education and experience, the medical staff repeatedly concluded that we were perfectly healthy. Furthermore, they felt our age was a positive. I was 26/27 years old when all this was happening, and my husband was 28/29. Both of us were medically within the ideal weight ranges and my menstrual cycle was extremely regular with ovulation. Moreover, sperm analysis showed to be normal, hence we had no reason to disbelieve what the doctors told us repeatedly.

Still, we were added to the waiting list for in vitro fertilization (IVF) whilst being comforted that it was unlikely to come to that. We ended up having three rounds of IVF and intracytoplasmic sperm injection (ICSI). With 38 eggs retrieved over the 3 rounds and sperm understood to be suitable/normal, you would think, things would be in our favour.

The devastating result was we were left with zero embryos across all rounds. A disastrous outcome. Results from the three rounds of treatments were astonishing to us and the medical staff on our case. Our case was labelled as unexplained subfertility and experts had extraordinarily little answers for us. The total time between the first visit to the doctor and the last consultation visit after the final ICSI round was about 5 years (2010-2015).

As previously mentioned, I decided to be happy at the onset. I chose to find peace and live my life well. This was significant because as the journey went on, I was exposed to more and more women and couples in the same difficulty. With this exposure, I noticed that many women, from all ages and backgrounds in this situation, were living in a world consumed by TTC.

Their sole focus was to get pregnant and deliver a healthy child. A great deal of joy from their lives seemed to disappear, and whilst I understood, I knew this approach would not work for me. This meant that although every failed IVF/ICSI round hurt and every year that passed without having a child was hard, it was not consuming us, it was not consuming me. My use of the term 'every year' is very intentional here because I didn't concentrate on it every month and cry when again my period came. There were months along the way where this was the case, but for the most part, this was not my common experience.

IVF/ICSI/IUI

In vitro fertilisation (IVF) and intracytoplasmic sperm injection (ICSI) are not for the faint-hearted. You will know this if you have gone through it. It may be something you will experience in the future.

It is commonly understood that there is a lot to process when using IVF/ICSI, both emotionally and physically, especially for females. Finance may also be an additional matter to work through depending on the situation and country of treatment. However, like most things in life there is no one shoe that fits all and experiences vary greatly.

In terms of the emotional, physical, and social aspects of these very invasive and draining treatments, I can say I was blessed for two very manageable rounds. I felt good throughout and didn't fully grasp why there was so much discussion regarding the hardships involved and why so many women complained about how difficult they found it.

Yes, the injections were painful, and the result was always shocking and heart-breaking, but all in all, it was not so bad. This great fortune of mine ended during the final round which began in autumn 2015. Without exaggeration, I can say it was one of the most challenging things I have had to go through in adulthood. Finally, I was able to fully comprehend the literature and the personal tales that discussed the devastating rollercoaster of said treatments.

It may have been the protocol I was on: Due to the disastrous outcome from the two previous rounds we had already undergone, consultants at the clinic decided on an aggressive and longer round, which meant that my body was battered and bruised by numerous injections.

By the final few nights, my eyes were streaming with tears from the sheer pain caused by every injection, and we were rapidly running out of viable injection sites on my body. These tend to be around the thigh area, glutes, or stomach, but there is only so much the body can easily handle from prolonged injections in the same areas. My body became sensitive and throbbed in pain.

Another major factor that complicated this round was that I had started a new job, this difficult IVF/ICSI round was happening during my initial probationary period at a new company. Management did not know my situation and I did not feel comfortable sharing it with them so early on, worried that I may not pass probation.

In the UK, these IVF/ICSI treatments involve a countless number of last-minute hospital appointments. Normally there will be a call from the medical team on your case, summoning you to another check-up, scan, etc., and this will happen multiple times without notice. You can imagine my stress, having to explain numerous, unplanned absences from work during my first few months with a new employer.

In contrast to that, during the first two rounds, I had been with an employer who knew about the situation. Thus, when I was absent without notice, there was no extra pressure and only well wishes. The experience of working somewhere where management did not know what I was going through and where I feared the potential loss of my job made me realise the blessing, I had had in the first two rounds.

That extra stress made my third round of treatment so much harder than I could have ever anticipated.

To add further injury after such a harrowing experience, it was another unsuccessful round. The final consultation meeting we had proved to be highly distressing, to say the least. After so much reassurance at the beginning of the 5-year journey, our consultant concluded that he did not believe this treatment (IVF) would be effective for us. He declared our case as 'the strangest case he had seen in 25 years of doing this work'. Talk about a kick in the teeth. I recall the feeling of numbness, of shock, of deep despairing pain and because of all that we knew we couldn't go again, at least not for a while.

Take a break when you need it

By January 2016, I knew that I was unable to continue with this for much longer and come out on the other side functioning well. I felt worn out, confused and hopeless, and so my husband and I decided to have a break for a few years.

I wonder if this is something you have done or are planning to do. I wonder if the idea seems absurd to take a break from trying to have a baby for as long as a few years. But this was the only way we could cope. I felt the effects of my body being filled with foreign and unnatural medication. I felt the effects of being prodded and inspected so often and so intimately. I felt the effects of disappointment after disappointment.

Taking a break for a few years was the gift we gave ourselves, for our health, our faith, and our marriage. This planned break lasted almost 4 years and I went from being 31 years old to being 35. This may freak you out if the thought of wasting those precious years sounds horrifying to you. I have zero regrets about this decision and would make the same choice again and again because my health, my happiness, and my marriage must come before my dedication to having a baby.

During this time, people did encourage me to take a shorter break, to avoid wasting so much time, that I was 'not getting any younger'. The only reason I was unaffected by these comments was because I was so sure about my decision. You need to give yourself a break when you need it and leave worrying about time or age to someone else.

The 5 years of TTC I described consisted of trying to conceive naturally, then having multiple tests, and finally 3 rounds of IVF & ICSI.

The only thing I chose was to be happy through it all.

When I would speak with other women who were also TTC, I was often taken aback by their level of knowledge and their immersion into understanding everything they could about this new world they found themselves in. In a stark contrast to that, my approach was to be proactive enough to seek treatments as quickly as I could but remain mentally and emotionally disconnected as much as possible.

I left it to the experts and took myself off the hook by not having to be so involved in every little detail of the treatment. This was part of my coping mechanism; it helped me avoid being overwhelmed. This is what I needed at the time.

I am not sure if you are more like me or, more like the highly involved and highly informed women, or possibly not yet engaged with any of this. You may be avoiding tests, possible treatments, and disappointments. Wherever you currently are, I strongly encourage you to choose your approach at each stage consciously and intentionally.

In the past year, I have tentatively started to re-embark on the journey of actively TTC. This has been a frightening thing to re-enter after such a long break, but my approach is a bit different this time, in how I physically and mentally engage with it.

This time around, my plan is to be so much more involved. To be in charge at each stage in terms of being fully informed and understanding my body and our case as much as I can. I feel I am more able to handle this now as I have had the required break, gained more strength and understanding over the years, and feel more equipped for this approach. I think it serves me better at this stage in my continued journey to motherhood. You may wonder if my age has influenced this change and I am sure it plays a big role, but if you were to ask me if I would do anything differently, my answer would be a no. My approach back then was what I needed at that time and my current approach is what I need now.

Tools I used to survive TTC

As I currently write this, it has been over 12 years since we first began to try for a baby. Outlined below are some of the key tools and approaches that saved me during it all.

The most defining factor and my saving grace in trying to conceive for all those years was deciding HAPPINESS had to come before MOTHERHOOD. Despite how much I want to be a mother, I know motherhood cannot be the only way a woman, a woman of faith in particular, can achieve happiness. This is contrary to popular belief and messaging from ourselves and society. Another thing I decided was more important than TTC was my marriage; you can read more about that in chapter 8.

One other coping mechanism and approach that worked extremely well for my husband and I was humour. This was not intentional, but it became our go-to. We found so much laughter in the ridiculous situation we found ourselves in. It is this humour that saved us emotionally and mentally through the ordeal. Please find laughter where you can because we both know the tears are plenty.

In addition to all that, the most effective way I believe I have been able to achieve happiness and ease through this is to continually focus on other goals unrelated to TTC. I cannot stress how important this one is because when you make becoming a mother your everything and fixate on it, the journey becomes so much more damaging to your spirit and life. For that reason, I continuously have so many goals related to business, finance, spirituality, travel, and more.

One particularly large ambition of mine for many years was to become a homeowner in London (UK) without a mortgage. Anyone living in London or a similar city can attest to the magnitude of this goal. My desire level, my why and my dedication to the goal, was intense and most importantly, it was unrelated to trying to get pregnant. Being occupied with this allowed me to pursue something other than a baby. It allowed my heart to breathe and stay centred as well as giving me a sense of control whilst feeling utterly out of control in my pursuit of parenthood.

Homeownership may not be your goal; it may seem insignificant compared to motherhood. But having other deep desired goals that are personal and important to you will make a huge difference in your ability to thrive and conquer whilst trying to become a mum.

Apart from having varied and specific goals, another important focus for me is the pursuit of balance. What I mean by this is the desire for me to have success and fulfilment in my life holistically. This love of balance, for me, stems from my belief and understanding that life is the current moment; we do not know what tomorrow brings, and so, I aim to be in a state of gratefulness, hope, comfort, and joy in the present moment, always and in all areas.

To achieve this systematically, I have been using a tool since I discovered it in 2015 when I started training to become a Personal Performance Coach (Life Coach). It is called the 'Wheel of Life'.

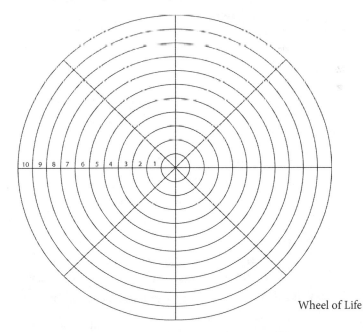

Wheel of Life

The way I use this is, at least once a year I assess my fulfilment level in eight key areas that are important to me. The key areas are faith, relationship (marriage), family, friends, career/ business, health, finance, and adventure/life experience.

I assess the level of satisfaction or fulfilment in each area by numbering them 1-10 (1 being low satisfaction and 10 being high satisfaction). My goal is to have as many 7s, 8s, and 9s in all areas on the wheel. If an area is 6 or below, it becomes paramount for me to work on that area without neglecting others. An area that usually scores low for me is family due to not having children or immediate family in the same country. But because so many other areas of my life are fulfilling, hopelessness and worry are inevitably lessened.

Why is any of this important? This is important, my dear sister, because you are a whole being made of many parts. You are designed to live life fully and purposefully, to take accountability and control of your life but with the knowledge that the result is always with your Creator.

I would urge you to try this activity and if you feel that some or many areas are lower than desired, re-focus your efforts in improving those areas to help you achieve more from your life. You deserve more happiness, so work for it in all areas of your life instead of focusing on your infertility trial. You were not created to be sad; permit yourself to live fully and purposefully and with genuine gratitude. This can only be achieved by deciding to want it, deciding to notice the blessings filled in your life, and working to grow that happiness.

But do you even want a baby?

I must stress that my intentional approach to choosing happiness without yet attaining motherhood should not give you the impression that I am not maternal enough or wonder if I want a baby. My maternal instinct has always been strong and yearning for motherhood has intensified by wanting to have my own family over the years.

If you feel overwhelmed by your maternal instincts, wanting to see yourself in your children, to give birth to humans that are part of you, part of the person you love the most, then, I am with you. I feel it too and I want that more than I can adequately put into words. However, I don't believe that if you choose happiness or pursue other dreams, you somehow don't want to be a mum, that you are giving up, deserting your child to be. This is far from the truth. You can want to be mum to the point where it physically and desperately aches, and still find the strength to find life enjoyable, joyous, full of adventure, and even fun.

I do not know how long you have been on this road. Many women find even six months on this road a harrowing experience, and my heart goes out to you if it has been long. With that understanding, you and I both know that your baby will not arrive a minute earlier than it is meant to, so why can't you find some light whilst you wait?

Permit Yourself

I hope you see that my journey so far has not been an easy one but nor has it been all doom and gloom either. The past decade of my life has been a beautiful blessing. This may be hard to grasp considering how much I have wanted—needed—to be a mother.

The decision to be intentional has played a pivotal role in allowing me to cultivate an approach that supported a positive outlook. This led to actions and pursuits that reinforced that outlook and created a life of light and beauty where there could have easily been so much darkness.

I wrote this book for you. I share my journey to get you thinking about your own, possibly from a different perspective. I know that my strength with this is not an accident. I know that my infertility struggle is not an accident. It was designed for me as yours was designed for you. Know that you too are strong. You can become stronger. Strong doesn't mean you don't cry. It doesn't mean you don't feel sad. It means that despite the sadness you continue with life. You find, grow, and experience joy and keep on choosing it every day, every month, every year for as long as you need.

Your vulnerability is strength. You are strong even when you cry at the sight of seeing your period arrive once again. You are strong even when you ache with pain, longing to hold your child that you must consciously remind yourself to breathe. You are strong even when you break down as you wake to realise it was all a dream, that you hadn't become a mother. You are strong through it all for as long as you do not allow this to beat you, to imprison you. You are strong for as long as you do not believe that your life has come to a standstill while you wait to be a mum. Life is now. Living it fully is your choice. I don't claim it to be an easy choice, but it is your choice. Permit yourself to live it.

CHAPTER 2

WOMANHOOD AND IDENTITY

W hat were your life dreams when you were a little girl? How about in your teenage years?

It is highly likely you dreamt of various and exciting accomplishments. Within that mixture of dreams, two big dreams were probably constant. Not only were they constant but also interlinked, you couldn't achieve one without the other (as a Muslim at least), and once you achieved the first, you automatically got the second, right?

What two dreams do I refer to? They are the dreams of being a wife and a mother. Additionally, unlike some other personal goals or dreams, these two dreams are often expected, both by yourself and society at large.

You expected to grow up, get married, and have healthy children. You may have had other dreams around career, travel, and various personal goals but they were likely in addition to being a wife and a mother, not without them. On the other hand, you may have had no other dreams or goals other than being a wife or a mother.

How does this happen, who created this expectation, and where does that leave you today? The expectation that women become wives and mothers is not new. It's been the most dominant position in which we have seen women for the longest time. It's the role in which we have seen women for as far back as we can recall in history. To add further emphasis on this expectation, many faiths including Islam promote and honour women within these roles. The Prophet (SAW) said, "… is your mother alive?… stay with her, for Jannah is under her feet" (Sunan al-Nasa'i, 3104).

The associated respect with said roles is far from a negative matter. For many Muslim women, these roles provide meaning, honour, and fulfilment that are unmatched. The issue arises when this expectation is not met for whatever reason.

Unmet expectations could be due to a woman not wanting it for herself. While this is still quite uncommon, especially in the Muslim community, it's fitting to mention that there are women who don't wish to be mothers for multiple reasons. Navigating such a choice in the landscape in which we have described has its challenges.

For others, marriage may be delayed or never occurs, and for others, like you and me, the sudden and unexpected reality of infertility has become part of our story. With this unplanned setback and the dream seemingly lost, we are left with the task of re-evaluating ourselves, our position, and our choices.

In that situation, the question now becomes where does the individual woman begin, and the identity attached to trying to conceive end? What happens to identity, the self and expected roles for the one struggling to attain motherhood?

I appreciate the odds are stacked against you. How you are reminded daily of your 'difference' to other women. How you feel that you have yet to join a very special circle—a circle open to all women, as long as they are mothers.

I know you want to be part of this circle. That it hurts to be banned and shunned from it. How at times it feels overwhelming, isolating, lonely, and a burden to bear. I understand and acknowledge your pain.

All this is totally understandable, but we must remember that your specific circumstances as well as your destiny—including your struggles to conceive—is part of a precise plan that has been specially formulated for you by your loving and wise Creator.

'…. And it may be that you dislike a thing which is good for you and that you like a thing which is bad for you…' (Quran 2:216).

It is incredibly important that I remind you here: the experience you are facing was chosen for you. Nothing about your experience is an accident. Nor is it a punishment. Nor was it ever in your control. The Almighty hasn't forsaken you. He hasn't created you inferior to other women. Nor has He made being a mum the totality of being a woman.

My dear sister, on this journey you must know in the core of your being, in the depths of your heart as well as logically within your mind, that He has a plan for you. That He did not make a mistake and He designed for you this journey as a way of achieving success, peace, and contentment, in this world and the next.

I know it is hard to accept and to give in to the notion that what is happening right now is happening for you. If you reflect on this, you will see the wisdom in some parts of it while in others, not so much. Regardless, I promise you that there is wisdom and a reason and design in this seemingly unfair, chaotic, and random test you find yourself in.

Identity

To manage the loss of a dream, unmet expectations, and all the elements stacked against you due to this trial, there are key aspects of yourself that require your protection: identity, womanhood, and self-worth. I am grateful that even in the darkest hour I refuse to ever doubt my identity, womanhood, or worth. Carving out your own identity and paying close attention to feelings and beliefs around your worth is something you need to do and redo often. This is to protect and honour yourself through it all so that you become and remain strong in the face of a test that has the capabilities of breaking you.

Womanhood and identity are difficult to navigate whilst on the journey of trying to conceive. However, you must start to regain and own your identity as your happiness and self-image depend on it. It's time to start dismantling the identity that you and the world assigned to women, and by consequence, to you.

Now is the time for you to create an identity for yourself that considers your situation, that can support a positive outlook, where happiness, success, and hope can live. Find it, create it, hold on to it and celebrate it. This means infertility cannot be your identity. I will not pretend that this is an easy task, but you must, I must, we must. Otherwise, we will not survive this world that is often described as a Man's world, but which can often feel like a Mum's world. A society where so much of the everyday seems to largely be catered to, for, and by mums.

Furthermore, have you noticed the destructive narrative the media keeps feeding us about 'childless' women? She's always batshit crazy! Harsh words, but they're true. It doesn't matter if the character has a health problem or her male partner has a problem or they have unexplained infertility, in just about every film or TV program I see about a couple trying to conceive, and it makes the woman/would be mum emotionally and/or psychologically unstable. She will often try and steal a baby at some point. She may seduce random men to get pregnant. Other times she's found being involved in strange things like black magic.

It astonishes me how the media continues to portray women who are not mothers as inferior, unstable, unlovable, and desperate. This all plays into the long-standing image of what society decides is a 'real' woman. It can, if you are not careful, add to negative assumptions or beliefs about your fertility, womanhood, or marriage.

The 'unstable' female characters I am talking about are fictitious characters made-up in films, but you have to be aware of the stereotypes that the media portrays, and determine for yourself an identity which you define, rather than accepting one that is pushed on you. My own identity involves seeing and knowing myself to be a strong, good, resourceful person. A person protected and under the care of her Lord. I see myself as someone of integrity and morals who treasures independent thinking.

These parts of me that I hold so close to the core of my being mean that it is impossible for me to feel worthless because I have not yet birthed a child. It makes it impossible for me to see my worth through my role as a wife or lack of worth through not being a mother. Separating my identity and worth from trying to conceive means that the outcome of my TTC journey doesn't affect who and how I see myself. Who and what I am and TTC are and will remain separate; it's this separation that is imperative for you to recognise and strive for in your own journey.

For most people, procreation is a natural and wonderful desire, and therefore the message of this chapter is not to ignore or diminish your desires to be a mother. You have a right to want this for yourself. You have a right to be confused by your situation. You have a right to be sad by the loss you feel. But your worth and identity should not be the casualty of this. They need to be built on a strong foundation that prevents you from wavering or buckling under the pressure that accompanies TTC.

This is a book to remind you that you are worthy. As much as it can sound a cliché, it is the truth. However, the caveat for this truth is that it must resonate as the truth for you. You must believe this so fiercely, that there is no room to think otherwise.

Questions and Activities for Chapter 2

Now that we have discussed in detail womanhood, identity, and unmet expectations, it is time for you to reflect on your ideas, beliefs, and thoughts around who you are and how you see yourself. Answer the following questions in your journal with as much detail and honesty as possible.

Q1. How do I see myself?

Q2. What is my identity?

Q3. How do I value my worth as I am?

Q4. What new perspective or belief can I adopt about myself and who I am regardless of what happens with my TTC journey?

CHAPTER 3

THE BODY AND THE PERIOD

We've discussed in detail the importance of reconstructing our beliefs around our worth, our identity, our womanhood, and now it's time to turn our attention to the body we live in. I wonder what your beliefs are about your own body and what you say to yourself about it. Is it harsh and degrading? Is it fair? Or is it one of love and appreciation?

Your body, like yourself, isn't responsible for what it goes through; it can only do what God allows it to do. Thus, the stark reality is that disappointment, anger, or revulsion towards it aren't fair or constructive.

Could we choose to honour our bodies? To be grateful and hopeful and in awe of how magnificent they are. Don't worry, I am not taking you on an airy-fairy speech fest about affirmations and self-love (although you may by all means go ahead with this if it's your jam). Instead, I want us to look at our bodies and analyse them with an objective mind. With that aim, let me give you my approach.

As much as possible, I ground my views about my body rationally. I focus on all the things I can do (like writing this book right now), because without my hands, my eyes, my back, none of it would be possible. This body is a gift from the Lord of all the worlds for me to use until I no longer need it. To hate it or be angry with it would be a disservice to this body and could potentially be a sign of ungratefulness towards He who created it.

Unfortunately, many women feel their body has let them down, that their womb has let them down. They feel that it has failed to do what it was created to do, but who decides what it does, the womb or its Creator? Every cell in our body does more for us than most of us can comprehend. Your struggle to conceive or carry a child to full-term doesn't mean the body has failed nor that your womb or any other part of you is a waste.

Once we can adopt the perspective of proactivity and the belief that everything is working *for* you rather than against you, you can look at your body through a different lens. You can learn to love it for all that it has done and continues to do for you.

My body, like my worth and identity, will not be degraded by this experience. My body was with me before any ideas of being a mum came and it will continue to be strong and flourish as I will.

The separation mentioned earlier is vital. You must separate the TTC experience from all other important parts of you and your life. What will you do to protect your body, in a similar way to your worth and identity, from becoming a casualty of TTC?

A woman's period is a strange thing on the journey of TTC. Large numbers of women in this boat develop a love/hate relationship with it. Love because without it, conceiving would be virtually impossible. Hate because its arrival is a brutal reminder and confirmation of no pregnancy for another month. Again, this is another thing you can take control of if you want to. You can decide how you see your period. I know having your period can be hard and it is ok to feel disappointed, but it is important to find the light—big or small—wherever possible.

'*We are not animals; we are not products of what has happened to us in our past. We have the power of choice.*' (Steven R. Covey)

I choose to love and honour my period because it is part of me and therefore, I have nothing short of love and appreciation for it. I also love it because for as long as I am menstruating, there is the hope of becoming a mum. How can I be angry with it for existing and showing up regularly, when without it the dream of motherhood would die? My dear sister, the time is now for you to reclaim your happiness, your worth, your identity, your womanhood, your body, and even your menstrual cycle. They all need you to protect them so that you can be happier and healthier for it.

What can you do today to reframe negative feelings about your body/menstrual cycle?

Write 5 ways you are grateful to your body/period. Keep coming back to this. It will give you that necessary shift when you need it.

Look after your body. Make it strong, both emotionally and physically. Work out, go for walks, eat well. Access services such as counselling to release trapped trauma or emotional distress.

Beautify your body for yourself. Smell good. Wear clothes that make you feel beautiful (in your home at least). Pamper yourself where you can with essential oils, massages, hot baths, spa days. Love this body!

CHAPTER 4

IN THE COMPANY OF GREATS & DELAYED PARENTHOOD

What are the requirements for being a woman? Do you fall short of such requirements if you are unable to conceive easily?

Does it feel like you're stranded on an island on your own whilst other women are busy popping out children as easily as changing their clothes? It can certainly feel like that at times.

As if you are left behind, whilst other women, other couples, graduate to the 'next stage' of life. Leaving you on the married but no children platform. Failing to match the expected path to grow up, get married, have children, have grandchildren, and then pass on with the legacy that is your progeny.

Some communities believe 'someone who leaves' children behind when they die never actually dies. They continue through their offspring. I understand how this can have you questioning your position in society, in your family, and what your future will be.

It's during times like these when it's crucial for you to catch your thoughts and create beliefs to support you instead of those that will harm your well-being. As discussed in chapter two, your Lord has not forsaken you and if not being able to conceive meant you were less of a woman then you would not be in the company of great women. Great women who have been introduced to us through our faith, which so many of us hold so dear.

Many of these women were the wives of prophets. Prophets chosen by God as messengers of the Truth. These great men and women from history that go as far back as to Prophet Ibrahim, were not tested with delay in parenthood because they were forgotten, inferior, or being punished with it. Neither are you and your husband.

These women had children at a later stage in life or were never mothers. Examples of these women include Prophet Ibrahim's wife, Prophet Zakaria's wife, Asiya (the wife of Pharaoh), and the mother of the believers, our beloved Prophet's youngest wife, Aisha.

The Quran directly mentions the topic of childlessness in the stories of Prophet Ibrahim and Prophet Zakaria. A line that never fails to make me smile refers to the response of Sarah, Prophet Ibrahim's wife, after angels informed her of her pregnancy:

'And his wife approached with a cry [of alarm] and struck her face and said, "[I am] a barren old woman!"' (Quran 51:29).

This makes me smile because I can imagine the scene so clearly: the lack of hope that preceded this outcome, then the joy at this news. The loss of hope of this ever happening for them is so clearly portrayed in Sarah's response. I also love this *ayah* because it shows how *my* situation is similar to tests experienced by amazing women in Islamic history.

We too are great women. And we need to believe this and permit ourselves to live a life that is nothing short of great.

Statistics show that infertility is experienced by 1 out of 7 couples in the UK, 6.1 million American women aged 15-44 (Womenshealth.gov) and 48.55 million couples worldwide (WHO, 2010).

There is comfort here, in remembering you are not alone. You are not the first and you most certainly will not be the last to experience this. Use this as fuel to strengthen yourself and to give your heart contentment as you navigate a purpose-filled life.

Statically speaking, you are part of a huge number of women and couples going through the same pain. The few examples given above also demonstrate the calibre of historic women you are amongst.

In everyday life you are repeatedly exposed to pregnant women everywhere (even the celebs seem to be at it) but the reality is, there are millions of women in the same boat as you. There are couples in the same boat as you. Some are older than you, some are younger, some married for years and others for a shorter period, women of all ethnicities and faiths and across all six continents.

Therefore, know with certainty that you are not alone, and although your circumstances make your fertility journey unique, the experience of infertility itself is not unique. There is comfort in remembering this and adding it to your toolkit to get you through when it all feels so isolating.

Benefits to delayed parenthood... what?

Everything in life has advantages and disadvantages, and infertility is no exception. Wait! Hear me out first, do not throw this book away just yet.

On a serious note, though, if you take the time to reflect and recognise the positives in delayed motherhood, you will see that there are many. Granted, you would in all likelihood give them up in exchange for a healthy child, but they are still pros that can genuinely make your life better, if you recognise and enjoy them without worry or guilt.

Listed below are some of the positives I have recognised and enjoyed over the past decade.

Freedom – The joy I get from having the freedom to do what I like, when I like it without worrying about childcare is golden, and so are simple pleasures such as being able to travel outside of term-time (unless you're a teacher, I guess).

Finance – Let's face it, raising children is not a cheap task. Whilst I don't encourage delaying children due to fear of poverty, it's nice to have extra financial security and freedom whilst waiting to be a parent. On the flip side, fertility treatments can be awfully expensive for many, especially depending on where you are in the world so this may or may not be relevant for you.

Pre-baby body – We know that many mums miss their pre-baby body (there is a whole fitness industry dedicated to solving this problem) but you already have that right now. Enjoy it, appreciate it, and strengthen your body because one day you may look back and miss what you have today.

Being a priority with yourself and your spouse – This is a luxury because most mums are focused on being a parent, and self-care and prioritising their wants and needs may seem self-indulgent. Try to enjoy it whilst you can.

No contraception – Most long-term contraception options are potentially harmful to women, with side effects for many. Being able to enjoy intimacy within your marriage without this burden is something to notice and appreciate.

Better preparation for parenthood – We know that parenthood is not something you study in a textbook or become perfect at. Nevertheless, there's a lot to say for personal growth which can aid parenting once you achieve it. For example, my personal growth throughout the years I have been TTC—emotionally, in my relationship, in my finances, and my confidence—makes me believe I would be a much better parent today than if I had fallen pregnant when I first began to try.

Do any of these benefits resonate with you?

What positives can you find in your situation for a better life now?

CHAPTER 5

THE MOST DIFFICULT QUESTION

This book is intended to be a resource for you to tap into when you need it. It's also meant to challenge and encourage you to consider a different way of experiencing infertility.

It pushes you to understand—and hopefully accept the truth—that the hardship you find yourself immersed in is not the end of your life. While this book encourages you to adopt a different mindset, it does so with the understanding that this will require a lot of bravery from you.

Bravery to have to experience, to read about, to ponder on, and to act on what is discussed. It is perfectly understandable to instead want to pause, stop and bury your head in the sand. I know the inevitable fear that is present in all parts of this journey sucks. I recognise the bleak outlook you see in your life and future. However, remaining in this state, with this limited mindset, does not serve you or those around you.

Whilst this reaction is understandable and exceptionally common, the fact remains: a passive and/or negative response to your situation is non-effective in most cases. I have seen first-hand clients who have increased their feelings of disempowerment and despair by ignoring what they face. They hope that by not knowing more or by just making *dua* it will all work out in the end. However, life experience tells us that this is not a recipe for success.

I spent a big chunk of my working life in the charity sector. For many years I worked in a charity where we educated local people (mostly women) about preventing or detecting cancer early through screening programmes.

These programmes included smear tests, mammogram tests (breast screening), and bowel screening. All three save lives. All three are generally harmless. All three are available through the NHS in the UK for those eligible. Despite all that, the obstacles we faced often were people saying they did not want to have these routine tests in case it 'found' something. Our response to them was always the same: We reminded them that it was unlikely that something sinister would show up (these were routine tests after all), and more importantly, if something was wrong, then it would be better to know. Not knowing or ignoring something does not make it go away. We informed them that at least if they knew, then they had the power and choice to do something about it. The earlier the better as well.

The same applies to you. If you are experiencing a delay in parenthood, whether this is a male, female, or an unexplained issue, the truth is that you are in that position. That difficulty is there. It is your reality regardless of how proactive or reactive you are about it. For the topic of infertility, ignoring it could mean avoiding initial tests, important conversations, and not exploring options in treatments.

However, if you are frozen by fear and confusion then this chapter will be particularly challenging to process. Nevertheless, it is vital for you to force yourself to take ownership of this experience.

Most of the content and key messages in this book were written for you with the assumption and hope that you will end up with your dream biological children. That this harrowing journey was designed for you before the gift and light of your baby. I pray this is the case for you. I pray this is the case for me. I pray this is the case for all of us.

Whilst this hope and prayer is important, this book would be a total disservice to you, to all of us on this journey, if we avoided the challenge of facing our truth. There is something none of us want to look at, consider, or accept but we must if we are to live and bring forth a good, grounded life.

What I am referring to is the question of:

What if I never have a biological child?

This question is confronting and hard and could be interpreted as thinking negatively, but it is important we face it head-on and sincerely.

Why is it important? It's important because making decisions, making plans, and exploring options can only serve us in a way that is healthy and long-lasting if they are based on reality. The reality we need to come to terms with is a balance between hope—that we will be given what we desire (a child)—and the truth that we may be given something else instead.

This difficult question will be met with horror by some people. One reason for such a reaction is the new age thinking around the idea of manifesting. Manifesting refers to the idea that one has the ability or divine power to create anything and everything one desires through positive thinking, visualisation, and through 'energy'. In many parts of the world, large numbers of Muslim women have also taken on such beliefs.

In Islam, there is an element of this that is controlled and balanced. It alludes to understanding information such as when Allah says, 'I am as my servant thinks I am...' (Hadith Qudsi 15). The meaning here is if one thinks Allah as stingy (*uadhabillah*), unable to give you what you desire (i.e., a baby) then one might get nothing as this is how he or she imagines Allah to be. In contrast, a better alternative would be to think well of God in His power and generosity.

Additionally, as Muslims, we believe that our *duas* are always answered. They are answered in one of three ways:

- By being given what one asked for
- Delayed to be given in the Hereafter
- By diverting an evil like it from us. (Musnad Ahmed,10749, Sahih Al-Albani).

I share all this as a reminder that Allah knows best. Our trust in Him (*tawakkul*) should not waver no matter the test.

Despite my intense desire for motherhood, my trust in Him has to be bigger. I felt it necessary for me to answer this difficult question after I was struck with the following ayah which moulded my outlook on infertility:

> 'To Allah belongs the kingdom of the heavens and the earth. He creates what He wills. He bestows female (offspring) upon whom He wills and bestows male (offspring) upon whom He wills. Or He bestows both males and females and He renders barren whomever He wills. Verily, He is the all-Knower and can do all things' (Quran 42:49-50).

Barren. That is the word that stuck with me. It stuck with me because it made me realise there are people—great men and women, from the past, in the present, and will be in the future—who are indeed barren.

There is no amount of manifesting, no amount of positive thinking, no amount of treatment that can change this if it's a part of their destiny. I asked myself why I would think that couldn't be me. And if it was, what next?

I asked myself the question to give myself a sense of control, a sense of peace knowing that I have considered all possible outcomes and that I have in theory planned for all possible eventualities and still keep choosing happiness, to keep choosing myself, regardless of the ending. Only God knows what will happen and none of the plans are guaranteed to pan out but by putting a plan in place, I can reduce anxiety for myself.

After TTC now for a long time and being a fertility coach for several years, I have had numerous conversations with women of all faiths and in particular the Islamic faith about their expectations for the future.

Most of the women declared they would without a doubt go on to have a biological child. On the surface, I do love and admire this thinking. It is bold and brave and maybe the truth. On the other hand, this resolve for a biological child 'come what may' causes me a level of concern.

It is complicated if one decides a biological child is their ultimate goal and a guaranteed outcome. There are questions we must ask ourselves to manage this goal and expectation:

- How do I know that to be the truth? Do I know for sure that it's part of my destiny?

- If this becomes the only outcome I care about, what might I sacrifice to get it?

- How secure are any of us that we are not in the group of barren people that the Quran refers to?

This is not to hurt or torture you. I have presented it to you in the spirit of truth, support, and rationality. I pray it serves you how it is meant to.

I once asked a client these questions. Her response was, 'the end'; there is no life without a biological child. Whilst I appreciate and understand her desperation in wanting a child, this sentiment and choice broke my heart. I caution you, my dear sister, against this staunch and depressing viewpoint on the matter.

You can aim to strive for a balance. I promise it can be achieved. You can take the necessary actions to have a child. To push yourself physically, financially, and spiritually to increase the odds of achieving your dream, and remain secure and comforted in the knowledge that your Lord is ultimately driving the ship that is your life.

As thoroughly discussed in chapter 1, you have control of *your response* to everything that happens in your life and the world. However, you don't have control over *what* happens. None of us do.

As Muslims, we leave the outcome to Him after we have put in the effort, with the belief that He knows best, and He is the most loving and the most merciful. Once we know and understand this, we can achieve the balance in hoping that we will receive what we desire while simultaneously knowing that there is a chance this may not happen. Therefore, if that is the case, how will you live, how will you love, what becomes of your life?

*

An activity for you:

Take a seat in a quiet spot and close your eyes.
It is your birthday today. You have turned 90 years old.
No biological child was written for you, so what became of

your life? What happy memories did you create along the way? What was the point of it all in the end?

If you could start again, would you do anything differently (that you had control over)?

If so, then MAKE that change now.

It seems I made a mistake and today is not your birthday, or maybe it is but you're not yet 90. You can decide now.

The question of what your life will be if you never have a biological child is exceedingly difficult to face, but it is also only as hard, complicated, or scary as we make it.

CHAPTER 6

EMOTIONAL SUPPORT

Infertility sucks. This daily battle is making you weary, and I know that because I am feeling it too. The pain that this experience is causing you is not something you can easily ignore. This is especially more difficult if the test has been prolonged for you. Anyone in this constant battle for 10+ years has my deepest empathy and love.

You deserve a guilt-free life

On the path to motherhood, many women become intimately connected to the feeling of failure which leads to guilt. I wonder if this is you.

I don't want it to be, but the likelihood is that you may have had moments of guilt. This irrational emotion which should have no place in your thoughts or feelings could be caused by a number of reasons.

You may feel guilty if you believe you are the 'problem', the one whose health is responsible for delaying parenthood in your marriage or delaying grandchildren for parents on both sides.

Other times you might feel guilty because you are being overwhelmed by the process and have let it control your life to the point you struggle to be happy internally and thus struggle with interactions with people. You feel you are making others uncomfortable or sad.

On the other hand, you might feel guilty because you think your 'bad' diet may be hurting your fertility.

For you, the guilt may stem from past experiences such as using contraception.

Or is it because you feel unable to support your husband better if he believes he is the 'problem'?

Whichever way you rationalise it, guilt has no place on the road of trying to conceive. It is an unwelcome passenger that is to be tossed out of the car as soon as possible. The only way you can address this in any meaningful way is to face it head-on; therefore, I want you to ask yourself two important questions:

Question 1 – *Am I or have I ever done anything intentionally to hurt myself, my body, or husband to cause infertility?*

I don't care what you think you have done in life thus far; you are not in control. I repeat, you are not in control of your fertility health nor were you in the past, so you did not cause this.

It's simply too harsh to berate yourself and steep in guilt because of the smallest choices. For example, you want to have coffee but have been told caffeine is bad for fertility. I am no doctor but, my God, have the coffee if you want it and it makes you happy. Please do not waste valuable energy allowing yourself to feel guilty over little so-called mistakes or choices you make now or made in the past.

We need to remind ourselves that women have fallen pregnant from a one-night stand or on their wedding night without doing anything 'good 'or 'bad'. Others have spent years doing drugs and worse and still regularly fall pregnant. I add these facts here to remind you that life is unpredictable. All experience of infertility you face now is neither meant as a punishment for you nor caused by your actions. Furthermore, we cannot know if anything is punishment, or not. A blessing for one person might be a trial for another person.

Question 2- *Does feeling guilty make you feel better or improve the situation?*

For most cases feeling guilty doesn't change the situation nor does it support you in building a healthier self, physically, mentally, and emotionally. I want you to go against habits of allowing yourself to dwell on mistakes. Question, challenge, and analyse your thoughts and feelings.

When you catch yourself feeling guilty over something that is outside of your control, ask yourself, does feeling or believing this add anything good to my situation? Does it make me feel better about my struggle? When the inevitable and honest response of 'no' comes back to you, then that is your cue to let it go.

Use that energy for something more productive. What can you do to change or improve your situation, even for the moment?

I know too well how it can chip away at you as the years pass by. It is, therefore, essential that you find ways to cope. Tools to help you individually and as a couple, survive emotionally and mentally through the dark days.

Below are some tools which may be helpful depending on where you are in the world. Many of the services or tools listed may also be available online and therefore accessible even if they aren't available in person where you live. Some services will have a significant financial cost, and others may be relatively low cost or even free. Again, this will largely depend on where you are in the world.

1) Counselling/Therapy

This is a great tool to unpack and explore your feelings around your fertility situation. It can be a safe space where you can discuss in detail your biggest fears, regrets, and worries with a professional trained to deal with and support people through their emotional and psychological needs.

It is a safe space to explore much of what is buried deep down in your mind or heart. Conversations in this safe space may focus on fertility or anything else you wish to discuss. For many, it can be a healing experience and you may come out on the other side stronger. This doesn't mean the process will be easy; it can at times bring out even darker days for some time while you unpack everything that lurks below, but healing is taking place. In the UK, IVF and other similar treatments usually have counselling offered alongside them.

This is usually the case whether treatment is via NHS or privately. It is not compulsory, but couples will be given the option to use it if they wish to. Outside of IVF treatment, counselling can be expensive, but many people and organisations are trying to make it easier for people to access. Therefore, good counselling is provided for free or at an exceptionally low cost through charities and other organisations. An online search should let you know what is possible within your budget locally or online. It is incredibly important that you check the credentials for individual counsellors you choose to work with to see they are reliable, qualified, and ethical.

2) Coaching

As opposed to counselling, coaching will focus less on digging deep emotionally and into the past, and more on the future and providing clients with tools to explore themselves and their situation. It facilitates opportunities for clients to formulate and execute a plan that allows them to go from where they are to where they want to be.

Areas of work on infertility for clients might include treatment options. Looking closely at available treatments and considering what's best for their situation. It can also include action steps around improving overall health in preparation for pregnancy, or financial goals for treatments, or other goals. It is especially useful for clients who are stuck and who feel they are not in control of their fertility journey.

Blocks around fear and confusion can also be explored in a different format to counselling. It is an action-focused principle and clients will work through agreed action steps between each session. The result is often measurable progress by the end of the coaching programme. Example action steps may include talking to a spouse about a specific topic, calling x number of clinics for initial consultancy, joining a gym, speaking to a family member about x issue, etc.

Typically, someone can access one-to-one coaching but, like counselling, it can also be accessed either as a couple or as part of a group programme. Costs can vary but one is often able to book a free/taster session with a coach to explore compatibility and price options. It is quite common to have sessions online, but some face-to-face options exist too. It is worth doing some research on it if coaching sounds suitable for you.

3) Prayer/Dua

Yasir Qadhi's book *The Weapon of the Believer* gives you an idea of how vital and powerful *dua* (supplication) and prayer are. As a Muslim, you may already pray often, whether that is *fard* (compulsory) or *nafl/sunnah* (recommended) prayers. You are also likely to make *dua*, but this can still be an overlooked tool in your systematic arsenal to cope emotionally, especially during hard times.

There is healing and comfort that is unlike anything else when you converse with your Lord. Begging Him to give you what you want as well as to strengthen you and grant you patience. Rely heavily on this tool. At times it can seem like your *dua* is not being answered, but remember that no *dua* is wasted. Learn the etiquettes of *dua*. Offer *dua* in your language as much as needed so you are fully connected. Familiarise yourself with the times when *dua* has a greater likelihood to be answered, like when fasting or during certain times on Fridays. Also, make night prayers (*tahajjud*) your best friend; it can provide much comfort and strength.

Here are some *dua*s that you may find helpful:

Dua for children and during hardship

'O our Lord! Grant us in our wives and our offspring the joy of our eyes and make us guides to those who guard (against evil)' (Quran 25:74).

'My Lord! Grant me from You a good offspring; surely You are the Hearer of prayer' (Quran 3:38).

'My Lord do not leave me alone (with no heir), while you are the best of inheritors' (Quran 21:89).

'My Lord! Grant me (offspring) from the righteous' (Quran: 37:100).

اللّهُمَّ إِنِّي عَبْدُكَ ابْنُ عَبْدِكَ ابْنُ أَمَتِكَ نَاصِيَتِي بِيَدِكَ، مَاضٍ فِيَّ حُكْمُكَ، عَدْلٌ
فِيَّ قَضَاؤُكَ أَسْأَلُكَ بِكُلِّ اسْمٍ هُوَ لَكَ سَمَّيْتَ بِه نَفْسَكَ أَوْ أَنْزَلْتَهُ فِي كِتَابِكَ، أَوْ
عَلَّمْتَهُ أَحَداً مِنْ خَلْقِكَ أَوِ اسْتَأْثَرْتَ بِه فِي عِلْمِ الْغَيْبِ عِنْدَكَ أَنْ تَجْعَلَ الْقُرْآنَ
رَبِيعَ قَلْبِي، وَنُورَ صَدْرِي وَجَلَاءَ

*Allaahumma 'inne 'abduka, ibnu 'abdika, abnu 'amatika,
naasiyatee biyadika, maadhin fiyya hukmuka, 'adlun fiyya qad-
haa'uka, 'as'aluka bikulli ismin huwa laka sammayta bihi nafsaka,
'aw 'anzaltahu fee kitaabika, 'aw 'allamtahu 'ahadan min khalqika,
'awista 'tharta bihi fee 'ilmil-ghaybi 'indaka, 'an taj'alal-Qur'aana
rabee'a qalbee, wa noora sadree, wa jalaa'a huznee, wa thahaaba
hammee.*

O Allah, I am your slave and the son of Your male slave and
the son of your female slave. My forehead is in your hand (i.e.,
you have control over me). Your judgment upon me is assured
and your degree concerning me is just. I ask you by every name
that you have named yourself with, revealed in your book, taught
any one of your creation or kept unto yourself in the knowledge
of the unseen that is with you, to make the Quran the spring of
my heart, and the light of my chest, the banisher of sadness and
the reliever of my distress. (Ahmed and Al-Albani graded it as
authentic.) (141)

اللّهُمَّ رَحْمَتَكَ أَرْجُو فَلَا تَكِلْنِي إِلَى نَفْسِي طَرْفَةَ عَيْنٍ، وَأَصْلِحْ لِي
شَأْنِي كُلَّهُ لَا إِلَهَ إِلَّا أَنْتَ.

*Allahumma rahmataka 'arjoo falaa takilnee 'ilaa nafsee tarfata
'aynin, wa 'aslih lee sha 'nee kullahu, laa 'ilaaha 'illa 'anta.*

O, Allah, I hope for your mercy. Do not leave me to myself even
for a blinking of an eye. (i.e., a moment). Correct all my affairs for
me. There is none worthy of worship but you. (Abu Dawud, Ahmed
& Al-Albani graded it as good in *sahih* by Dawud)

لَا إِلَهَ إِلَّا أَنْتَ سُبْحَانَكَ إِنِّي كُنْتُ مِنَ الظَّالِمِينِ.

Laa 'ilaaha 'illaa 'Anta subhaanaka 'inne kuntu minadh-dhaa-limeen.

There is none worthy of worship but You, glory is to You. Surely, I was amongst the wrongdoers. (Al-Tirmidhi & Al-Hakim declared it as authentic and Al-Thahabi agreed with him).

(*Sahih duas from Fortress of the Muslim by Sa'id Bin Wahf Al-Qahtani*)

4) Journaling

Journaling is a powerful tool that costs as little as the price of a notebook and pen. Journaling consists of writing about whatever is on your mind. Your worries, excitement, fears, and anything else. You can do this daily or whenever you feel the need. It can be extremely helpful in connecting to and managing your emotions.

The best way to approach it is to not think about what you will write, but instead, allow yourself to pour on to the page without judgment. Don't worry about how it sounds or even if it makes sense. Your goal is to dump all your thoughts and feelings onto paper and get it out of your body. There is a healing and a calmness that can be achieved from this that is unique and special.

Keep your journal safe if you don't want anyone else to read it so that you can write freely knowing that what you say on these pages is between you, the paper, and God.

Write as little or as much as you need, but the longer the better. For example, 10-20 minutes is useful if that is all you can manage, especially to begin with. However, if you're able, journaling for longer periods will allow you to access deeper feelings you may not be aware of. This gives you increased information about yourself and your state of being, as well as possibly unlocking ideas and opportunities. It can genuinely give you greater strength, heal wounds, and manage anxiety.

'Journaling is an outlet for processing emotions and increases self-awareness … and expressive writing is a route to healing—emotionally, physically, and psychologically' (HuffPost 2017).

Some people prefer to journal in the 'notes' section of their phone or using a computer, but there is evidence to suggest that writing with pen and paper provides something vital and important.

Similarly, there is the argument that 'writing removes mental blocks and allows you to use all of your brainpower to better understand yourself, others and the world around you', and that journaling allows you to 'clarify your thoughts and feelings, know yourself better, reduce stress, solve problems more effectively, resolve disagreements with others' (Psychcentral 2020).

I have journaled on and off for a few years but have now been journaling regularly for about a year. I find the activity a source of release. A space to get my thoughts and feelings out without burdening anyone else with them. It also allows me to figure out my deepest fears and desires. It is also where I find solutions to the issues, ideas, and thoughts I am working through. I really do feel that it is aiding my health and well-being.

I urge you to try this if you haven't already. Use it on days when the noise in your head gets too loud. When you feel like you could explode, when you feel you have so much to say but are uncomfortable or unable to say it to others.

5) Support groups

Numerous support groups exist in forums online for women struggling with infertility. They are generally for people of all faiths and backgrounds and may or may not be suitable for you. You might also want to find out if real-life support groups for this topic exist locally. Furthermore, there is an increasing number of support and information-packed accounts on social media for all women, including for and by Muslim women.

Such groups, whether online or in real life, tend to be run by women in the same situation or who have been there. Stories are shared and members use the space to lean on each other, to answer questions, and to share emotional struggles. These groups often serve as a reminder that you are not alone, and lasting friendships can be built from them. Accessing this type of help is worth considering, but if you feel that the atmosphere and/or discussions are incompatible with your values or needs, then you can always leave.

6) Friends, Family, or Spouse

You will have friends and family that can be a source of comfort during difficult times, whether or not they have children. It may be unlikely that close friends and family have directly experienced infertility or are qualified professionals to deal with such matters. As a result, they are unable to provide the same level of support or solution you could receive from a counsellor, coach, or support group. Nevertheless, these people are a huge asset that many women like you and I can use.

They love you and want the best for you, so although they may not always know the best thing to say or do, there will be individuals who you can speak with frankly and use for support on the days where you need that extra emotional aid.

At times, it's important to have clarity on what you want from these conversations and be able to express that to others. Too often, people can go into problem solving mode and friends and family members who feel they know you might suggest ideas and/or possible solutions. This is not necessarily negative but if what you need is a shoulder to cry on or an outlet for a rant, then let them know so they can provide a listening ear.

You should also find a way to check in on your spouse. At times when you need a good cry or to share your worries with him, then do so. But since he is also in pain regarding the same issue, being sensitive to his needs is important.

7) Physical health

Aid your emotional and mental well-being by taking ownership and control of your physical health. Get it in optimum condition through exercise and other activities. Engage in workouts that are suitable for you based on your aim, interest, and body type. If you are inexperienced in exercising, start with basic research on beginner options to get fit. This could include sports, swimming, or going for a walk. Other workout routines for cardio or strength training are also important.

For me, a 30-minute walk 3-5 times a week and strength training (lifting weights) as often as I can are my go-tos. I strongly believe that these forms of exercise help me mentally as well as giving me the type of physique that I want (strength instead of skinny). There is also masses of evidence and research backing up the benefits of strength training for women concerning hormonal balance and mental health.

There's endless information through books, the internet, TV, and people we know to educate ourselves on the best nutrition to accompany good exercise. With effort and research, you can discover the best foods to better support your fertility.

I encourage you to check out the above tools to help you thrive through your situation, whether you access them now or in the future. You can also do further research to identify what is most suitable and compatible for you based on your needs, your location, and where you are in your 'trying to conceive' journey.

And remember:

> 'What is meant for you will reach you even if it is between two mountains. What isn't meant for you won't reach you even if it is between your two lips' (Arabic proverb).

And:

> 'You were given this because you are strong enough to live it' (naturalfertility.com).

CHAPTER 7

DEALING WITH SOCIAL PRESSURES

The previous chapters of this book have provided you with information and tools to strengthen your mindset; to help you understand and come to terms with your personal situation.

The remaining chapters in this section shift towards a focus on social pressures and interactions with others. This includes practical tools to help you overcome difficult exchanges with family and friends, especially in groups or large gatherings. Examples of such situations include dealing with pregnancy announcements, baby showers, Mother's Day, offensive comments, and other pressures from family, friends, and the wider community.

This book encourages you to get to know yourself, your triggers and your emotional state deeply so you can face infertility head-on. One thing I wish to impress upon you in this section is the significance of finding a way to manage your reactions to pregnancy announcements, baby showers, and other social pressures.

Dealing with pregnancy announcements

One of the many struggles that a woman or a couple facing fertility issues will encounter regularly is pregnancy announcements. Announcements from friends, family, colleagues, and even celebrities. Your reaction to such announcements will depend on your emotional state and what is happening with you at that moment.

Whilst it is important to avoid stifling your feelings, it is also extremely important that you do not allow emotions of shock, anger, or jealousy to override your rational thinking or peace. It can be easy to fall into the idea of 'it's not fair' when you see other women fall pregnant easily. You can be especially susceptible to this if the one who has become pregnant is someone you deem 'deserves' it less. Someone you feel is less 'maternal', less prepared, too young, too unhealthy, etc.

This thinking is simply flawed, no matter how rational it may seem. Firstly, for this to have any form of accuracy, one has to believe that life is 'fair' according to *your* judgment, and we all know that is not how life works.

Secondly, and more urgently, it is dangerous and unproductive to question the decree of your Lord, to allow yourself to think that someone else is less qualified to be a mum because *you* deem their situation to be inferior to yours.

If you spend years TTC, you will certainly witness others in your immediate circle or otherwise fall pregnant 'overnight' whilst you keep on waiting. However, you must remember that no one is ever given someone else's gift nor is anyone given someone else's test. It is not always easy, but you must find the strength to be supportive and genuinely happy for others. This will protect your own heart as well as protecting others from any harm or unkindness from you.

The 'why me' response was a fundamental reason why I struggled to find a connection with the online forums and support groups. The 6th pillar of faith in Islam is to 'believe in Al-Qadar', predestination, whether it be good or bad. Thus, it proves difficult for me to question what happens (or is destined) in my life as well as what happens (or is destined) for others.

I know that even though you know all this, you will still struggle with these 'why me' feelings. Please view these pages as a gentle reminder rather than a harsh judgment. Balance and rationality are essential. The religious aspects of this book are meant to serve as an addition to the practical tools and tips on coping with the heart-breaking experience of infertility. The two aspects combined work effectively together to help you navigate this journey, to (hopefully) find it a bit easier.

Here are three tips to manage your feelings and thoughts following a pregnancy announcement.

Flee to Allah

Please trust me on this one. Regardless of your level of *iman* (faith) or whether you pray or not, let this be the first thing you do. Make it a habit. Whenever you feel negative feelings, including anger, find a quiet spot, and talk to Him. Seek your needs directly from your Creator, sincerely and passionately asking for ease, protection, and support. If you feel that your *iman* is currently low, just know that despite that, your Lord still hears you and can still lighten your burden.

Gratitude

Gratitude is an effective tool to change your negative state to one that is positive and constructive, and it can aid better health and happiness. Make a list—whether on paper or just mentally—for all that you are grateful for at that moment. Do this slowly and reflect on each point. Both Islam and modern-day beliefs attest to the increase of goodness and blessings by being grateful. Allah says, 'If you are grateful, I shall give you more' (Quran 14:7).

Analyse to understand what you are feeling

Are you sad for yourself but happy for the other couple? Or are you feeling that it shouldn't be them/her, but you who is pregnant? There is a big difference between these two. Don't vilify yourself but be curious about what is going on. If you ever find yourself feeling that it shouldn't be her, that it should be you, then try to process the feeling. Remind yourself rationally that what she has was always meant for her, she didn't take anything away from you. Your blessings and trials are for you and hers are for her.

Dealing with baby showers

Another subject that has become increasingly popular in both Muslim and non-Muslim communities, especially in the west, is something called a baby shower. A baby shower refers to a party or gathering for the expectant mum, especially for her first baby.

Such parties may be big or small, women-only or both genders. It is an opportunity for family and friends to celebrate the mum to be and the new child before it arrives. It is a time of joy for many, when close friends and family provide gifts, play games, and enjoy the occasion.

I will not discuss here the permissibility for baby showers in Islam. You are free to do your research if the topic is something you come across or must consider in your community. For the purposes of this book, I will treat it as an idea, an event you may or may not attend. Whilst a baby shower can be a lovely occasion, it can prove challenging for those struggling to conceive or have a child. If you live in a part of the world or are in circles where baby showers are common, it's useful to prepare your response in advance.

You want to avoid being triggered every time and having to work through the emotions and possible personal conflicts at the height of the stress. Be proactive as opposed to reactive.

If these occasions bother you and affect your emotional well-being, then being honest with yourself first is paramount. Please move away from judging yourself harshly; you have the right to find this type of gathering hard and should not feel bad about it.

It's also important that you are honest with the mother-to-be who you likely know and love. By being honest, you avoid causing confusion or misunderstandings about not wanting to go or having to force yourself to go even when it hurts.

You can speak with her to explain that although you are happy for her, it's a sensitive gathering for you to attend.

We must hope that a conversation such as that, approached honestly and sincerely, will be taken well. Most women close enough to want you at their baby shower love and care about you. If they know your situation with TTC, they too are likely to want to protect you. Hence, they will understand your reservations about going. There should be no pressure from you or others to attend.

On the other hand, it's important to mention that you may not at all be affected by either circumstance mentioned above. If this is the case for you, then that is a blessing and a great space to be in. However, we have a different issue to deal with in this scenario.

The concern here becomes dealing with expectations from others. In circumstances like these, people often *assume* that you are affected, sad, or jealous. The result then becomes that those within your circles may delay or hide their pregnancy announcements and/ or avoid inviting you to baby showers.

Their intentions are usually to protect you, but as everything else discussed within the pages of this book, you want to take as much lead and ownership of this situation as possible. You can thank them for their consideration but reassure them that they don't need to make assumptions about your feelings or fragility. Let them know how you feel. Be clear that they don't need to hide happy occasions from you and leaving you out may be hurting you more.

At this point, it's worth briefly mentioning that as Muslims we do believe in the evil eye. Sadly, some might worry about this as a possible threat, but having frank and sincere conversations can prevent or resolve unnecessary misunderstandings. More importantly and effectively, it is valuable for us all to use the *duas* and or *ayats* directly from the Quran to protect ourselves and others including Surah al Falaq, Surah al Nas and Ayat ul Kursi.

Mother's Day/The Word Mum

Pregnancy announcements and baby showers are tough to deal with for many women struggling to conceive but another difficulty you might face is Mother's Day. This is a widely celebrated occasion, and the media, especially social media, extensively covers it during the lead up to it and the actual day each year.

In recent years, I've found this day increasingly more difficult and therefore try to avoid it as much as I can. I especially want to recognise and give my heartfelt empathy and understanding to you if, on top of struggling to be a mum, you have lost your mum too.

There is a special form of pain that this situation causes because there is without a doubt a tremendous suffering in losing a mum and not being able to be one yet. I know this pain well, and at times, to the point where even the word mum/hoyo/mama can be a cause of discomfort and hurt. I don't deny that Mother's Day and possibly the word mum in general will be a struggle for all women TTC, but I do think that there is another layer of pain for those of us without our mums as well.

Unfortunately, I don't have tips or words of wisdom to ease your pain on this one, but the way in which I've been able to deal with this unique pain myself is to: 1) acknowledge, understand and accept my feelings, and 2) remind myself that, in a similar way to infertility, I wouldn't have this test if I was unable to cope with it.

CHAPTER 8

AN AWESOME MARRIAGE

L et's start this at the beginning, shall we?

Before marriage and the expected kids, there was you and you were intrinsically enough. You were created and then informed by your Creator of your purpose on this earth when He said, 'I have not created the jinn and mankind except to worship me alone' (Quran 51:56).

You and I were informed here that the only judgment of hierarchy in the eyes of our Lord is based on piousness. Not parenthood, not wealth, not ethnicity. This means you have been given all you need to fulfil your purpose on this earth. Everything else is a bonus. It should be enough and a comfort to know that fulfilling our purpose is the goal. On top of that, we were then given blessings upon blessings so that we would recall and would be grateful.

The outcome of this knowledge should mean knowing yourself, loving yourself, and being confident that you don't need a husband nor a child to be valued. You can want a husband and a child as further blessings to your life, but you don't *need* them to be alive or to fulfil your life's purpose. You are a miracle. Scientists believe the probability of you being born in the first place is 1 in 400 trillion. (The Epoch Times 2014). You are the creation of the Almighty. You are enough.

The facts in the statements above and the reality of the world we live in is so contrasting it is heart-breaking. As humans, in societies, we decide what is important, how things should be, and often this is far removed from what we are taught in our faith, what was intended for us by our Maker. We fail to follow the divine laws and structures we were so graciously given, which creates much more suffering in this world than necessary.

One example of this, is that women's worth has for a long time been judged and determined through the titles of wife and mother. This is even prevalent in most Muslim countries and communities. An unfair and damaging stigma is largely placed on women in most communities across the globe regarding infertility. The World Health Organisation puts in the following way when explaining the stigma associated with infertility:

'An inability to have a child or to become pregnant can result in being greatly ostracized, feared, or shunned, may be used as grounds for divorce and will often justify a denial to access any family traditions. Disproportionately affecting women, the burden of disease is often assumed to be the fault of the woman...' (WHO 2020).

The cruel and unfair landscape described above and discussed in other chapters is not your problem to place too much attention on. The world cannot convince you that you are not enough until you accept it as truth for yourself.

To accept and embrace this position is a choice. I know you are probably sick and tired of being told what you believe or do, or think is a choice, but it is. Not enough of us challenge the programming and accepted truths around us to decide what works best for us.

If you take nothing else away from this book, I pray you take that. This is how to cultivate self-love and strength. I don't ever claim this to be an easy task; to choose a response that benefits you in all situations, even when it goes against what you have been taught from your environment, education, and expectations, is definitely not easy, but it is essential.

The second piece in this puzzle is your marriage. If you are a Muslim woman struggling with infertility, I assume you're married. This is not 100% always the case as demonstrated by the 1 in 5000 personal account in chapter 10. However, this chapter is for the married but childless women. I don't know for how long you've been married, how your marriage came about, or how it currently is, but the key message here is that the marriage itself is an independent entity.

I wonder if you have looked at your marriage in this way before. Marriage, like yourself, is enough as it is, or at least it can be. Marriage can be a safe space, a place of growth, support, and vulnerability. Your husband could be the person who knows you the most out of all the people on the planet, including your parents and siblings. Your marriage can be something that you choose to be grateful for daily by the amazing blessings provided through it and the blessing that it is. There are many men and women who want to be married, but a delay in marriage is their trial for this stage in their lives. This is not your test, so how can you find a way to enjoy that marriage right now?

Your marriage and 'trying to conceive' become the same for you when you merge them. By doing this, you set yourself to struggle considerably more than you might need to on a journey that is already arduous. Similar to linking your identity and self-worth to your TTC journey (as warned about in Chapter 2), by making your marriage reliant on the outcome of having a baby, you devalue it as well. An alternative is to separate the marriage and TTC. They mustn't be interlinked in your heart and mind.

See image for demonstration.

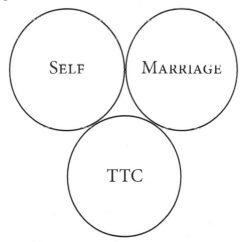

1) Ask yourself what the value is in separating the 3 parts.

2) Start to visualise in your mind a physical separation between all 3.

It may be useful to work through some ideas in a journal and complete the following or similar statements for yourself.

– I am enough as I am because ....

– My marriage is sufficient and enough as it is because...

– TTC is a valid part of my life that I can pursue without damaging myself or my marriage because ....

The next step is to create or enhance the honour and appreciation your marriage needs to be given. Begin by outlining and clarifying to yourself what you want your marriage to be. What does it look like? Feel like? What activities can you and your spouse do together?

How do you navigate TTC as a team? I urge you to give yourself and your husband permission to give this marriage its due rights and honour. It is a gift to love each other and be accepting of each other with or without a child. You need to know and recognise that this is important and possible.

What now? What to do once separation between the 3 parts has been achieved and the importance of honouring and enjoying your marriage is accepted and desired?

The next stage can't be accomplished alone. Instead, the layout, aim, and design for your ideal marriage should as much as possible be created by both yourself and your spouse.

What to do if one side is unwilling to do this or the connection and the open, honest conversations are difficult? In these cases, the advice on focusing on what you can control comes into play once again. You can't control how someone else (even your spouse) deals with this test, so whilst I encourage you to find the way to work together on this, it's not always easy.

Psychologist and relationship expert, Shelley Sommerfeldt encourages you to 'process your feelings first'. Once you are aware of where you stand and how you feel about the matter (any matter), it becomes easier to communicate with your spouse.

Furthermore, Sara Malik, NLP Master Practitioner who specialises in working with Muslim couples with fulfilment and intimacy in marriage, strongly suggests that you "allow yourself to be open and vulnerable when talking about your feelings, desires and most importantly needs".

Where you start, how you approach it, and how far you go with the below suggestions depends on where you already are in your marriage. Keep in mind that a good marriage doesn't just happen. It takes work, and certain aspects can be difficult or awkward. The hard work and discomfort are all worth it because the rewards are plenty. Building a strong foundation in your marriage is non-negotiable if you are to thrive through the challenges of infertility.

I'm not a relationship expert or psychologist and there are many resources to help you and I work towards better marriages and relationships. With that in mind, my suggestions below on how to honour and enhance fulfilment within your marriage are based on my own experience and the experiences of other women who are also TTC. Some points may seem like common sense but are still worth noting for the benefit of us all.

Prioritise it

Make your marriage a priority. As a couple, you must decide that your marriage is No. 1. A happy and fulfilling marriage doesn't happen by accident, and it doesn't continue to be fulfilling especially with added challenges—such as fertility. Thus, making it a priority will help immensely.

A way to prioritise it is by blocking outside voices—those of cultural norms or social pressures—that may weaken or confuse it. By prioritising your marriage, seeing its beauty, you are less embarrassed by the lack of children from it. By making it and each other a priority, you will continue in good standing during difficult spots along the way, keeping you feeling secure at times when you feel the most lost.

Have FUN!

Marriage and adulthood don't always need to be so serious, even for a Muslim couple, regardless of what society and certain cultures may think. Marriage (if we are blessed enough) is for the long run, and this is the person you are to spend eternity with. I don't know about you, but I need some fun in that kind of relationship. Fun for you as a couple and fun for us may be vastly different, but does that matter? No. What matters is that you have the kind of fun that makes sense for you and that you see value in. This is of utmost importance especially when something as heavy and serious as infertility is in the mix.

Have an adventure

Like having fun, choose to have adventures together that create a partnership, memories, a distraction, so that you become stronger and happier individually and as a couple.

Types of adventures can include business projects together, learning new skills together, traveling the world together, building and executing interesting new goals together, spiritual adventures together such as Umrah or Hajj, or establishing charities together. The point is to choose to seek joy and excitement through it all with what you already have.

Become each other's rocks

Men and women are at times quite different. Due to that difference, at times (not always), each gender feels more comfortable confiding in or being supported by someone of the same gender.

This book is a prime example. I am writing this book for Muslim *women* experiencing infertility. That is because I am her and thus, I feel I know her better. I am not writing it particularly for the Muslim male in the same boat.

However, for your marriage to survive infertility, you and your spouse must be able to support each other. You both want the same thing. You both feel the sadness and pain. Therefore, know and recognise that you and your husband need each other immeasurably to get each other through it. Be each other's rock. Cry to each other when needed. Share each other's feelings at any given point. Hear each other's worries and reassure each other.

No one can know either of you as deeply as you know each other, so cultivate the relationship and space where you can be there for each other during the hard days. Lord knows there are hard days. Through it all, you can survive if you become each other's rocks.

Reclaim intimacy

Sex is one of the most natural and pleasurable experiences that has been given to both males and females. It is something that is encouraged and rewarded in our *deen*, to the point where it is considered a charity (*sadaqah*) for both parties.

I mention this because anyone who has struggled with trying to conceive knows that soon enough intimacy can become all about ovulation dates and schedules followed by pregnancy tests. If you make that the aim and focus of intimacy within your marriage, you (the couple) can make something that should be a form of connection, joy, ease, and enjoyment into something cold and calculated.

It gets filled with pressure and guilt, and whilst optimising ovulation dates, etc. might be useful for you depending on your situation, it can't be the only reason for being intimate. It's healthy and appropriate for you both to reclaim this part of your relationship from TTC.

Have tough conversations

Part of building a secure partnership filled with all the things mentioned above also means having to have some uncomfortable and painful conversations at times. The key ingredient that will protect and reinforce your marriage is communication, communication, communication.

It's as straightforward but as hard and as uncomfortable as that. The No.1 tool in your marriage for all things on TTC and everything else comes down to talking and communicating. From this, trust is built, understanding is achieved, closeness is experienced, and solutions are found. The type of communication referred to here goes beyond mere talking or exchanging information to something so much deeper.

Conversations that require rawness and honesty. They provide the ability to discuss and work together through fears, options, obstacles, and needs.

What to do when your spouse won't communicate about this issue? Sara Malik gives these top tips to overcome this obstacle:

1. Let your spouse know 'why' it's important for you to communicate and set a time and place when you are both free and able to talk calmly.

2. If things are difficult between you, work on your relationship. A good place to start is to cultivate a relationship that is rich in gratitude and respect. The more respected and appreciated you both feel in your marriage, the stronger your union will be, giving you the ability to get through these sensitive times together.

3. Have your own support circle and encourage your spouse to do the same including working with a professional coach or counsellor together or apart if suitable. Having support outside of each other makes supporting each other easier and allows for better communication and understanding.

4. Plan and book in the time to talk about the big issues. Set a date and time and put it in your calendars, a light reminder on the day of the appointment is helpful in case either of you have forgotten or are avoiding hard discussions.

By normalising and making honest conversations regular, you can create and make your marriage a space that is a refuge, where you both feel secure and loved. It also becomes a place where answers are found, and plans are made.

Problem-solve together

An extra concern that you may face in your marriage is the issue of the husband's role in the TTC journey. I worked as a coach for several years specifically on infertility for Muslim women. I also spoke with women from all different backgrounds in researching for this book. In my conversations, a topic that cropped up more commonly than anticipated is the husband delaying or refusing tests in the initial investigations or during treatment. Clients I have worked with have expressed distress in not knowing what to do when their husbands don't want to take even the first steps to get the issue looked at through testing.

Reasons given by some men in talking with their wives have included 'it is not a big deal' and that 'there is no rush'. Others have suggested the act of providing semen analysis is *haram*.

Regardless of perceived reasons or intentions, the result is the same: the woman, desperate to be a mother, is left having to overcome extra pressure and solve a further issue.

As it is already the case, most of the responsibility for tests, treatment, or lifestyle changes often fall on the shoulders of the female despite what the health issue is or if there is an identified health reason at all. With all that in mind, it breaks my heart that women around the world must also shoulder the burden of researching, convincing, or justifying a lack of involvement from their male partner.

This is a particularly sensitive problem to address or work through if infertility is thought to be a male issue within the relationship, potentially affecting his masculinity.

Society often thinks that infertility lays with the woman automatically. Statistics show this is not the case (see below).

> Fertility experts agree that, on average, 30% of the cases of infertility they see can be attributed solely to the female, 30% solely to the male, 30% a combination of both partners, and in 10% of cases the cause is unknown. (fertilityanswers.com)

It can be even more challenging for men to consider the reality that a health issue with fertility may lay with them. This can cause increased fear, driving the male to delay taking steps forward in discovering the 'truth'.

Many wives want to also protect their spouse in a very trying time, but this can often be detrimental to her mental or physical health and/or her self-esteem. Infertility is hard whether the cause is considered male, female, or unknown. But you are not required to be a martyr, so find a way to work together through this.

To build a safe/judgment-free and confidential space within your marriage is paramount. A place where fears and problems are faced head-on, together, rather than both suffering in silence. A place to avoid tiptoeing around each other. It is enormously difficult, but it has to be the goal so that you both find strength within your marriage, and ultimately survive this ordeal, both as a team and as individuals.

CHAPTER 9

WHAT FRIENDS AND FAMILY NEED TO KNOW - YOUR MESSAGE

This chapter is designed as a tool for you to learn how to articulate to your loved ones what you need them to know and how you need their help with this difficulty.

Provided are 7 key messages aimed to help them reconsider their actions and thoughts so they can better support you and your husband on this road.

You can use these key messages for your personal awareness, to help you begin to identify which, if any, of the issues affect you or might do in the future, and how you can build boundaries that better support you.

Many of the messages address mistakes, possible offense, or harm that, for the most part, is born out of ignorance and lack of awareness. Still, the issue of dealing with social pressure and thoughtless comments becomes yet another problem for us to address as women facing infertility. It's a factor we need to face head-on to protect ourselves. Like other aspects of this journey, by confronting this with honesty, we can have more of our needs met.

Most importantly internal happiness, true self-acceptance and trusting in Allah (swt) and the process, all discussed throughout the book, will aid your ability to cope with unwanted comments and views from the friends and family.

With all that in mind the 7 following messages are directed to the friends and family, but really it's also here to serve as reminder for ourselves as well. Also provided following some of the messages or issues is a possible response you can use in that situation. Ultimately the responds will depend on the person and situation but the key message from me to you here is that you do have a right to respond in whatever way is reasonable to you. You have nothing to be ashamed of.

Principle 1– Respect is a basic requirement

A young woman I spoke with before I started writing this book said it best when she said, "The minute you get married, your womb and period cycle become the world's business".

This quote says a lot and demonstrates the lack of respect family and friends show to women or couples trying to conceive, as well as any recently married couple. Family, friends, colleagues, and other people in their respective communities need to be sensitive to the fact that women TTC don't need this type of invasion or questioning.

It's perfectly acceptable in many circles for women to share information or updates on their menstrual cycles, pregnancies, or babies. While this is useful and acceptable for many, it's not always the case for every woman and it may not be the case for a woman trying to come to terms with and understand personal and private obstacles to parenthood.

Probing or thoughtless questions such as 'what are you waiting for?' or constantly staring at her stomach and enquiring if she is expecting is not helpful, to say the least. There could be countless reasons for 'delay' in having a child. Furthermore, questioning her physical appearance is not acceptable. She might be tired, hormonal, bloated from IVF injections, or be on her period, so please be quiet on this one. Leave her be. Let women be. A woman knows her situation and what she is doing. If the relationship is close enough, she may share her fertility struggles with you, so be patient, be respectful, and let her lead any relevant conversation. Also, if she is or becomes pregnant, I am sure you will know in due course.

Your potential response: "Sweet of you to ask. I will let you know if there is anything to update. How is...?" (Change the subject firmly and politely).

Principle 2– Stop with the miracle babies

How many are you on now? I mean how many miracle babies have you been told about where the couple were married for 15+ years, gave up all hope only to discover they were pregnant. I have personally lost count of such stories and I don't think I had asked to hear about one of them.

Friends and family mean well with this one. The aim is to increase hope and motivate us, but it may not accomplish what they expect. Sure, this will be a comfort and a reminder of some of Allah's grace and power, but for many, it is not helpful.

Additionally, at times such stories are like Chinese whispers and it becomes hard to decipher their accuracy.

Your potential response: "I don't know about all that, but we make *dua*" or can simply say "I hear this a lot and it's actually not helpful for me, so do you mind if we don't talk about this right now" and change the subject.

Principle 3– Don't be a doctor (unless you actually are :))

This one's is for the lovely friend or family member, often advising couples—or more commonly the female—about miraculous herbal teas that guarantee pregnancy.

It isn't limited to teas either. We get told to listen to specific Quranic verses for certain amounts of times or sexual positions that will do the trick. It all needs to stop. As well-meaning as all this is, it's usually unhelpful, invasive, and incorrect.

The truth is they want to help, and we appreciate the sentiment, but they are unlikely to know more about the reproductive system, complicated medical barriers, and or God's plan. All that this type of advice causes then is confusion, misplaced hope, wasted money or time on something unlikely to be effective.

At times, this kind of advice may be harmful to your health or well-being.

Your potential response: "Thank you, I've started my own research".

Principle 4– Take your own advice

Another big suggestion freely dished out to couples trying to conceive is 'why don't you just adopt'? Again, like the rest of the suggestions, this is not helpful nor is it unique. You are likely not the first to suggest this and whilst adopting is an option for many (discussed further in part 2), it is not helpful when friends and family who themselves have never adopted or discussed adoption throw it at couples trying to conceive.

Your potential response: "We are exploring all options. Adoption is something that can be positive which many people could consider. Have you ever considered it?"

Principle 5– Don't belittle their blessings

"A couple without children are just roommates. A child is what makes a family".

"You must do everything you can to have a child because children are the *only* joy in this world".

Both statements have been said to me in the past. It still shocks me people think this is appropriate or helpful for a couple struggling to conceive. What is the aim behind such comments? I sense it's a way for making the childless couple/woman understand how important having children is. *We already know.*

My dear sister, I am sorry if you have been told these words or similar in the past. I am sorry for the hurt that was caused in your heart and the peace that was robbed from your mind.

Your husband is not your roommate. Re-read chapter 8 if you need to. Allow the words and messages in this chapter to penetrate your heart so that you can find joy and contentment in your marriage. Be able to recognise it for the blessing and beauty it is.

If the only joy in this life were children, then God would have or will give you them; the time He delays parenthood means there must be more. He wants more for you and from you in this life and for the next, so find that joy, demand it, and work for it.

Your potential response: "A marriage without children is still a blessing and we are good, but thank you for your thoughts".

Principle 6– Follow their lead & ask questions

Some women or couples will want to discuss and share information with you regarding their TTC journey. They may also want to seek help from you in terms of advice or otherwise. It's usually best to take a cue from them. If they want to talk about it then you need to fight your discomfort in the situation and be there for them fully.

Do they need a solution, do they need a listening ear, do they need a shoulder to cry on?

Family and friends, need to find the strength to help them through this personal and terrifying maze that they have no map for. If the woman or couple open about their struggles, then ask them what they need, ask questions, and check in to enquire how they are, what has developed?

Feelings can change often and it's not always easy to know when they want to talk and when they don't. Don't be tempted to guess but instead ask them.

A close friend of mine did just that. She was expecting at the time of this conversation and already had children. She told me to inform her anytime I felt sad about hearing so much about her children or her pregnancy. We had a very open and loving conversation that gave us both permission (especially me) to share easily and openly about the struggles, questions, or requests that could develop whilst we were having vastly different experiences of starting a family.

What my friend did well was not assume that I would automatically be sad or unable to support her in her pregnancy because of my struggles, nor assume that I should just be fine either.

She checked in and asked me to speak with her when and if my feelings ever changed. This is so powerful. This is not as easy for women/couples who are not as open about their journey, but if the relationship is close enough or secure enough, you might still be able to have a conversation with them. The aim is to not assume anything and try to avoid making comments that could cause more pain.

Find the courage to ask questions such as 'what do you need from me', and 'would you like to talk about anything related to the situation?' Let them know that you are available for them so they can reach out when and if they need it. This means more than you realise.

Principle 7– Become their cheerleader and keep an open mind

You have to put aside your individual or cultural beliefs about marriage, children, and women if your views don't support the happiness of the couple. Help them seek opportunities for themselves and their future with or without children. If you haven't gone through fertility challenges, or even if you have, their journey and personal experience are different.

They need breathing space so they can unpack their experience and build something that works for them out of it. I must stress that this is not about you. It doesn't matter if you agree or yourself would do any of the choices they make when starting a family. You have to support them in their decision, regardless of what they choose.

This life is precious and being as content and as happy as possible within the boundaries of Islam is something, we should all strive for, so support them in their options and bravery.

Sometimes happiness is about creating a life others may not understand; it takes special/brave people to go against the grain and create a picture that is of their own making even when it is uncomfortable. Family norms, cultural pressures, and/or worrying about what others will say are not what they need to be thinking about. They need to be brave, open-minded, and solution focused. You have to try to do the same for their sake.

A special message from us (couples trying to conceive) to all you wonderful and special friends and families who want the dream for us: we see you; we see your sincerity, we feel your *dua*s and we love you. You aid our strength.

THANK YOU.

CHAPTER 10

STORIES OF THE BRAVE

Sister Amina: "To those who have miscarried – I may not have my baby in my hands, but I am a mum and so are you if this has happened to you".

***

This chapter is dedicated to the voices of the brave men and women going through infertility. In their words, they share their experience and struggles as well as providing you with words of advice. They are in my shoes. They are in your shoes.

The shoes might fit each of us differently by our individual and circumstantial differences, but they're the same shoes. As a result, you might see yourself, your story, in one or more of the stories in this chapter. I hope it erases all ideas of being alone. I hope it encourages hope. Please include these brave men and women in your *dua*s.

*All names have been changed to protect the identity of the lovely people who shared their stories.

Story 1

Name: Asia / Age 27 / TTC–2 yrs.

I think every girl just has this idea in their head of how marriage is going to go. That perfect fairy-tale dream of a grand wedding, a happy marriage, and then 1 year later, you are magically and happily pregnant with your first child. I mean that is what seems to happen to everyone else, right?

It is not until you face infertility or the struggles of TTC that you realise this dream is exactly that: a dream. I mean, for example, I married my dream guy *Al'Hamdulillāh*, we had a fantasy start to our marriage and then *Al'Hamdulillāh* we got pregnant 1 month after our 1st anniversary (I know dreamy so far). I'd been trying for about 10 months as I came off the pill to avoid hormone imbalance. But unfortunately, that is where my dream all stopped. My pregnancy had so many problems, including medication that can affect the baby from growing, etc. So we ended with a sudden emergency at the hospital. I lost my baby at 13 weeks. A miscarriage, my baby deemed as never living and just a 'product of conception'. It was devastating and life-destroying for myself and my husband.

I for one have never had physical pain to compare this to, and, well, the emotional pain has scarred me for life. Having to go through labour pains, water breaking, and then birthing your tiny baby took its toll on me and my husband. The loss tested our marriage, and it was no longer a dream. We were at a point where we were not sure we would work any longer and it was hard to admit that to each other.

After our initial loss, I went into a crazy whirlwind of depression mixed with the need to try again for another baby. I pushed my husband into trying before he was ready and I was obsessed with ovulation tests, sex during my fertility window, testing days before and after my periods. I became a TTC zombie.

After my miscarriage, I had a lot of pain in my ovaries and was given an ultrasound to check my uterus and ovaries. This was when I was finally diagnosed with PCOS.

I'd been tested 3 times before by blood and was always told negative. I'd been worried about PCOS because I'd watched my sister and cousins go through it and had prayed that I also didn't have it. Turns out I did, alongside my diabetes and weight, all factors that went against my chances of successfully getting pregnant again. I tried to get fertility appointments and we got booked in only to be cancelled a week before due to my BMI.

This is when I decided to have bariatric surgery abroad to help all my comorbid illnesses and *In'Shā'Allāh* conceive again. It's been nearly 2 years since I started TTC again and I've put my fertility journey on a new route so that I can finally get what we are all wanting: a healthy baby in our arms to call our own *In'Shā'Allāh*.

I found it difficult trying to find a community to fit into. The TTC/infertility/miscarriage community that isn't Muslim offers the real emotional support that you need, but it then becomes difficult because you aren't getting the religious aspect. On the other side, religious gatherings, people, dismiss emotions and just pushed you to have '*sabr*'.

The Asian community shunned me, and I was lost. I found friends online who are Muslim through an Instagram blogger who made a Facebook group, but this group didn't fill the void that our women needed. I and Amal talked about it for ages (she was one of the ladies I made friends with) and then she took the step to make our own Facebook group and make it more interactive. I joined her as admin, and we started Muslimah Infertility Support. *Al'Hamdulillāh* we then made an Instagram account and we've been just reaching out to as many women as we can in our community. We hope to provide a safe place because we didn't have that for a long time.

To all the women reading this, I make dua that you all have your baby one-day. Ameen.

Story 2

Name: Amal / Age 28 /TTC– 5 yrs.

It all started when I hit puberty; I had irregular periods. Didn't think anything of it. I was happy that I never had periods.

No monthly bleeding, yay! I didn't realise the severity of it, which is why I never got myself checked.

Only after a few years, the weight piled on. I went from a trim size 8/10 to a size 14/16! I went to the Doctors and they blamed my studies, saying that it was stress.

I persisted, told them time & time again that it was something else. After 3 years, I got diagnosed with PCOS. Again, I had no further knowledge and kept getting fobbed off.

It didn't worry me though as I thought I'd never get married. I thought "who's going to marry me anyway?" due to PCOS and my weight.

Fast forward. I got married alhamdulillah. We have been trying for over 5 years, & still nothing. I lie to myself, saying that I'm not the issue, when in fact, I am. I lie to myself, saying that I don't want kids, when in fact, I do.

My heart yearns to be a mother, yet I am never there. Some days I feel so alone. I don't speak about my troubles. But since making our Instagram page (Muslimah Infertility) I realised that there are so many othr women out there who feel the same way.

I have hope that, *in sha' Allah*, one day I can share all the love I have to give to other people's children, with my child. But for now, my nieces and nephews will have to do.

Story 3

Name: Lola /Age-29/ TTC -2 yrs

On the path to motherhood

You know, no woman prays or imagines that she would be faced with fertility challenges. I mean, growing up we take it for granted that once we get married, pregnancy follows automatically. I have faced quite a few challenges in my small years of existence but absolutely nothing prepared me for the struggle of trying to conceive.

Waiting month on month, hoping that perhaps I would get lucky the next month is both physically and emotionally draining. When you now finally hear from your doctor that the problem— the reason that your family hasn't multiplied—is you, it will take all the strength inside of you and special grace from your Maker not to crash completely.

When I received this news, barely months after undergoing surgery to remove a disturbing cyst (and you know what this does to you? It gives you hope that "finally, the problem has been removed"), I crashed literally. I wept so hard and I couldn't stop the tears from flowing. I kept on asking why. What have I done wrong? Haven't I been through enough pain already? But soon, I was able to get myself back together with the help of my ever-loving and ever-optimistic husband, and I started asking the questions that mattered.

I had to tell myself that crying or driving myself into a sad state would not rectify the situation. I told myself that I just needed to be strong for me first, then look at the bright side of life and all the stuff I have going on well for me.

It's been a little over two years of marriage and I'm optimistic on the path to motherhood.

Story 4

Name: Khadijah/Age 29/TTC– 9 yrs

This has been a hard battle, and for a long time it did feel as if everyone else got to receive their gifts, but I was 'forgotten about'. I know this is not the reality but that is how I felt. I also questioned my worth and felt life was 'boring' without a child.

To further complicate our fertility issues, I suffer from a condition called vaginismus. This means I suffer from 'painful spasmodic contractions of the vagina in response to physical contact or pressure, especially during sexual intercourse' (Oxford Dictionary).

My condition made everything about trying to have a baby more difficult for a long time, but in recent times, I have found much relief in herbal and alternative medicine which has improved my condition.

I am much more positive and proactive about TTC now, and I also do strongly believe that it will happen when Allah wills, whether my circumstances are against it or for it.

To manage the stress, I changed a lot of my focus on it in the last few years as I found that being idle was making it worse, so I refocused my energy on work and studies as well as being proactive in understanding my body and fertility through alternative treatments.

We are open to accessing IVF and may consider going abroad for it, but my husband is still a bit reluctant on having tests so we will need to do that first. I also want to avoid IVF and all the extra ultrasounds and injections if possible so this will only be a last resort for us.

The main thing I can advise another sister in the same situation is to keep busy and productive. Seek knowledge. As cliché as it sounds, focus on finding yourself and your passions. Increase your dua and istighfar. Get involved in something that excites you and your purpose.

Story 5

Name: Fatima/Age 32/TTC–N/A

Being 1 in 5000

I was sixteen and was yet to start my period, something all my friends had. Naturally concerned, my mum took me to visit the doctor. I didn't think much of it, I assumed I was most likely a late bloomer, or the doctor would give me some medication because all girls have periods, right? Wrong. After some medical tests, I was diagnosed with a condition called MRKH Syndrome. MRKH (Mayer-Rokitansky-Kuster-Hauser) syndrome is a rare congenital disorder affecting 1 in 5000 women.

In summary, I was born without a cervix and uterus and had the lower third of my vaginal canal. Contrary to what people initially think, penetrative sex is possible. Girls with MRKH do go onto have satisfying sex lives. Often girls will require assistance in stretching the vaginal canal, either through surgery or the commonly used Dilator Therapy. Genetically I am female, my external body is the same as every other female. I have functioning ovaries and fallopian tubes; however, I do not menstruate and will never be able to carry a pregnancy.

Being told this at such a vulnerable age was incredibly difficult. I felt my heartbreak, a physical ache. I was an adolescent being told I would never have children, I was different, I wasn't like my peers. I wasn't going to grow up and be the woman society told me I would be or expected me to be. The woman Islam ranks so highly: a mother. I felt broken, embarrassed, ashamed, and alone in this trial I was now facing. I felt like a failure even before I had begun.

My diagnosis left me questioning everything—my identity, my faith, my role in life, my purpose. If I couldn't have children, what good was I? Would I ever find a man who would accept me as I was, who would be willing to make the sacrifice of having his children for me? Why me? I became very isolated, lost any sense of self-worth, and confidence I had, and my mental health was heavily affected.

Coming from a background where topics such as sex, periods, infertility, or even feelings, are rarely spoken of, I spent a long time trying to deal with everything predominantly alone. I bottled up my feelings and thoughts and rarely spoke of it, thinking one day they would all go away. They never did. Eventually, I sought out therapy and I truly cannot emphasise enough the difference this can make.

Living with MRKH is a daily struggle, particularly as I have gotten older. Every new pregnancy announcement brings with it sadness. As happy as I am for couples experiencing pregnancy, there will always be a part of me that will feel sad for myself, and grieve for the child I will never carry but always thought I would.

Knowing I can't carry my child, or even try fertility treatments, knowing I will never see my stomach grow or experience that 'pregnancy glow', I will never feel my child kick, I will never know what it feels like to have a mini-me, will always hurt. I'm not sure if the pain will ever go away. However, with time I have learned to manage the pain and accepted that I am allowed to grieve, I am allowed to feel sad. Feeling this way does not mean I lack patience with Allah's will or I am ungrateful for my life, it simply means I am human.

MRKH brings with it many difficulties, whether it be the psychological impact, the pursuit of a relationship/marriage, sex, infertility. There are so many aspects of it, and it is a never-ending journey. With time I am coming to realise not being able to have a biological child of my own does not define me as a woman, nor does it reduce my worth. I am learning to love myself and show myself compassion, recognising the strength I have. Everyone is tested, some are tested with children, and others with not having children.

As Muslims, we believe Allah does not burden us with more than we can bear, and admittedly there have been numerous occasions where I have felt all of this to be too much, questioned whether I would make it—is there light at the end of my tunnel? However today I am sitting writing this and sharing part of my story with others. I've joined social media to raise awareness and share my experience; I never thought I would have the courage to do so.

For anyone in a similar situation, I would strongly suggest reaching out. You don't have to face this alone; you aren't alone! There are people out there who will relate to everything you're feeling, people who can offer you support and a shoulder to lean on.

What does the future hold for me? Unfortunately, IVF Surrogacy is not an option as a Muslim woman, womb transplants are in their early stages and I am uncertain what the Islamic position is. The only option available to me is adoption. For now, I am finding myself again and what it means to be 'me' and trying to let go of the negative feelings I carry. I am not those four letters that I let consume me. Yes, MRKH has its place in my life and it is a part of my identity, but it is not the 'be all, end all' of who I am.

Story 6

Name: Husnera/Age-28/TTC-4 yrs

It took me two months to 'get pregnant' when we first started trying to conceive. Without knowing it though, I quickly miscarried under the guise of a period. It wasn't until the bleeding returned a few days later that I had my HCG tests show a rise in hormones. Within a week, the hormone dipped, and a miscarriage was confirmed. Once again, 2 months later, I again conceived without knowing until I bled profusely and abnormally heavy for 2 days, then it completely stopped on day 3. A test confirmed pregnancy, but once again, within a week, the plateau in my hormones confirmed the pregnancy too would be unsuccessful.

This time, 7 weeks in, the bleeding returned, and it only stopped intermittently. For another two months, I started to bleed clots. I was advised by a gynaecologist, that I would need a hysteroscopy and D&C. This was cancelled on the morning of surgery by a doctor because of the implications such a procedure may have on my fertility. Instead, I was prescribed progesterone to resolve the bleeding. Within a month, the bleeding subsided but my stress levels were at their peak because it meant I would be trying again, and I didn't know what to expect. My GP referred me to the fertility clinic and over 2 years, I had numerous blood tests, scans, ovulation tests, trying Clomid in varying strengths, which all started to impact my mental health. I was finally referred for IVF. In secrecy, I awaited my first appointment with the consultant.

Once accepted for IVF, I consulted an Islamic scholar who advocated this option, and we went ahead. Like pregnancy, the impact of the treatment differs for all. I had no difficulties with the hormone injections; the extraction was uncomfortable, and I was bedbound with painkillers for about 24 hrs, but that was probably the worst of it. In comparison, my friend who was going through it at the same time however suffered from typical pregnancy 'symptoms' from the first day she was injected.

In the end, I had few eggs that were fertilised and only two lived to be returned to my womb as embryos. It was a difficult concept to process. I chose not to discuss it at all with friends and family and asked my mum to await any news if and when there was any news and I pretended I was not doing anything differently. My friend however chose to disclose her treatment with her immediate family and in-laws. I share these contrasts to show either way of managing treatment is fine. The one thing we both focused on was being stress-free, and healthy nutritionally in the lead-up and during the process.

One advice I was given by a friend who attended a talk by a leading fertility consultant was to put everything into reducing stress levels as a factor to help you get pregnant – whatever that is. I made a note in advance of what triggers and what reduces my stress levels so that I could start managing this.

Despite being successful in my IVF pregnancy, I opted not to discuss the process openly due to anxiety. Even today, with a one-year-old, it is only something I discuss openly on the topic of fertility issues, and when speaking with people on a personal level and as a means of hope. But the way I look at it, as I did before opting for IVF, it is nothing more than a mere step in my journey to motherhood. If you are struggling with fertility and it is an option for you, grab it.

The Males' Perspective

Story 7

Name: Hussein/Age 27/TTC–5 yrs

I always thought getting pregnant would be easy. I never knew there was so much more to it, especially for my wife. Temperature checking ovulation, fertile days. Not to mention the mental health side of it. The community makes you feel so alone. It sickens me how the community shuns those that are struggling to conceive.

I am a firm believer that Allah gives, and have hope that He will give us our blessings one day. It's heart breaking when I see my wife cry after hearing pregnancy announcements and knowing that it's not us. Knowing that my words cannot comfort her.

I feel it affects our women the most as society has drummed it into everyone's head that women should be able to have children with one click of their fingers. The only advice I can give to brothers out there going through the same thing is to be there for your wife. Don't tell anyone what's going on. Let her speak when she is ready.

Story 8

Name: Younus / Age 38 / TTC– 11 yrs

The main thing that many men brag about is how many children they have. Being married to my gorgeous soulmate for a long time and not having kids with her is hard. I have a blessed marriage, but we are missing little ones to make it complete. I try not to think about it most of the time and I place my trust in God.

I realise me and my wife are not the only ones going through this. Our families and friends feel the hardship also, as I see it in their eyes every time I play with my nieces and nephews.

One option is adoption, but do I really want to raise a child that isn't my flesh and blood? I don't know, to be honest. Most of us men don't talk about issues like mine, so I don't really talk to anyone about it. It's even worse when you meet new people, and you start asking each other questions. I always try to avoid speaking about family.

Now and again, you come across a total bonehead who, when he finds out I don't have children, will make silly statements like 'what, no lead in the pencil'? I can usually shut them up right away with my own silly remarks, ask silly questions to get silly answers, I guess.

But on a real note, God willing one day I get to experience what it's like to be a father, watch their first steps and for them to speak their first words and so on, children who can carry on my lineage. I want to raise good men and women when the time is right. I feel I would appreciate the blessing of having children which I have noticed a lot of people seem not to be aware of. Till then I'm still grateful to God for blessing me in every way and won't lose hope that one day, *in sha' Allah*, it all works out.

Story 9

Idris / Age 28 / TTC - 4 years

When I think about our TTC journey, I have always had this thing at the back of my mind that maybe I wouldn't have kids because I have a family member that couldn't. Therefore, our struggle was not a surprise to me at first. My only thought was, I hope I'm not the one that's stopping us because I know how badly my wife wanted children. At first, I dragged and delayed getting the test done for a while. I tried to ignore the situation, but once I did the test, it turned out, I was ok.

I felt terrible for my wife because I didn't want her to feel like she was the one stopping us. I do sometimes ask myself, how can I want or be upset by something I never had? We have now been married for four years, and in those four years, we have had time to build our relationship and chase our dreams and be in a better place financially so when a baby does come, we can be in the best place. Us getting pregnant is not something that weighs heavy on my mind, but I know it's what my wife wants, so I hope we can one-day make it happen *inshaAllah*.

Part 2

Treatment Options

TREATMENT OPTIONS

Parts 2 and 3 of this book are all about options. Options available to you and your spouse for treatments and the alternative ways in which you can grow your own family.

No parts of the information within this section are advice from me or a push towards a specific direction; but rather an opportunity to give you the details on what is possible, and available so that you can take next steps to design the best future you can for yourself.

In Part 2, I focus solely on fertility treatments available at the time of writing this book. The Islamic ruling on each treatment is also included. However, I must remind you this is not a book designed to discuss Islam and its rulings on matters in any detail. Rather, an attempt is made to lay out basic rulings to ascertain which treatments are considered to be permitted, 'halal', or forbidden, 'haram'. It leaves the responsibility on you to do your research, which may depend on the source of your Islamic information. There may be differences of opinion on some topics, hence I urge you to follow up with your own research where needed.

Something else to consider in reading through this section is that the information provided is largely based on England, United Kingdom and some from the US. Although most of these treatments are generally available worldwide, the exact procedures, timelines or costs will vary greatly. It's paramount to also familiarise yourself with differences in services if relevant. In England alone, for instance, there is quite a bit of variation and you need to check what is available locally. This is usually decided by the local Clinical Commissioning Group (CCG).

Cost of treatments is something that is included here as a guide and to provide some insight, but this is something that will be vastly different across countries and dependent on the year you are possibly seeking treatment.

Furthermore, much of the figures used here are according to the National Health Service (NHS) in the UK. There are also numerous private fertility clinics across the country and their specific treatments and cost will differ. Similarly, in the US, fertility treatments will be paid either privately or through health insurance. Health insurance for IVF and other Assisted Reproductive Treatments (ART) will depend on employer, state of residence and other factors. Everything included in this book is merely a guide, a starting point for some and in accordance with information available in 2020/21.

Treatment options

IUI, IVF & ICSI

The first set of treatments discussed are intrauterine insemination (IUI), in vitro fertilisation (IVF), and intracytoplasmic sperm injection (ICSI). I have grouped them together because although there is some variation between all three, there are also similarities between them.

IUI – This treatment is considered one of the more straightforward options for fertility treatments, in terms of procedure. It's successful for many couples and it's more affordable than most other treatments.

The procedure for IUI consists of sperm being placed directly into the woman's uterus. This is designed to replicate natural intercourse but by placing sperm directly into the uterus the chance of fertilisation is increased. It is considered a more natural alternative to IVF and some couples may choose this option if the issue of infertility is unknown yet or sperm is lower in volume or has mobility issues.

The 'best' sperm in terms of mobility is selected to be inserted into the uterus. This is done by using a speculum and a catheter to place sperm beyond the cervical mucus barrier to assist healthy sperm to fertilise eggs.

Following several ultrasounds to determine the growth of follicles, the woman is injected with medication several hours before the session to mature the egg and time ovulation.

The average cost of a complete IUI cycle is currently about £350 - £1,000. (Human Fertilisation and Embryology Authority, (HFEA UK) but can go as high as £1,600, according to the NHS website. In the US, the price range changes from $500 up to $4,000 depending on the medication, monitoring and blood work, and insemination (fertilityIQ.com).

Success rates for IUI are hard to determine and are influenced by too many factors. If you require further information, please refer to the websites cited across this part of the book.

IVF – This is probably the most common and most well-known fertility treatment. Some couples access this treatment following one or more rounds of IUI. It's often tried before using ICSI but that depends on the needs of the individual couple.

Your consultant will be able to advise you if and when IVF is suitable for you, if you want to consider it as an option.

Here is a summary for you on the IVF procedure:

Following some initial tests, you will be placed on a personalised protocol for your IVF cycle. The exact protocol is decided by your consultant and medical team. If the case is considered to be 'complicated' in any way, then several consultants or advisors within the same clinic can look at your case to develop the best possible protocol for you.

Each protocol will vary in length of time, exact medication, and how it is administered. Generally, all IVF procedures will include injections and specific medicines for treatment. These are delivered directly to your home or you are advised to collect them.

Once required medication and injections are with you, you are given a clear set of instructions. For example, this includes instructions to keep medication in your home fridge at a specified temperature. You are then given the go-ahead to begin treatment by injecting yourself once or twice a day for a period of time depending on the length of protocol.

There are different sizes in needles and injections are advised to be in the abdomen or thighs. If you struggle to inject yourself, you can get help from your spouse or anyone else in your circle who you feel comfortable with and knows your journey.

Whilst having daily injections at home, you will be given several appointments at the clinic. At these appointments you will have ultrasounds to track hormonal changes, follicle development as well as other checks. Appointments are usually booked last minute, and attendance is essential as changes in your hormones, uterus, and eggs occur daily. IVF is specific and rigid, which means you have to be thorough in following instructions precisely and attending each appointment.

Towards the end of treatment, you are asked to inject yourself one last time at a specified hour with a different medication designed to trigger ovulation. Following this trigger, you attend the clinic with your spouse at a specific time.

At the hospital, you will be prepared for surgery and sedated to have your eggs retrieved. The number of eggs collected varies greatly. Some women have 2 eggs retrieved whilst others have as many as 12, 15, 18 or higher. During your surgery, your husband will be asked to go to a different area within the clinic/hospital and provide a fresh sample of semen.

Once eggs are retrieved and sperm is collected, the two will be placed together in a laboratory dish for fertilisation to happen. The next step is a phone call to you from your consultant within 24 hours or at an agreed time to inform you if any eggs fertilised and if there are embryos available from the treatment.

If there are healthy embryos, you will be scheduled to go back to the hospital where you will have 1-2 embryos placed into the uterus. This follows two weeks wait to see if pregnancy has occurred. If the pregnancy test after the two-week wait is positive, it's a successful cycle and you continue with the pregnancy similar to any other pregnant woman. For health reasons, it's mostly advised to have no more than 1 embryo implanted, with a maximum of 2, dependent on factors in each case.

Mistakenly many often assume multiple numbers of embryos are implanted so more babies can be conceived per cycle, but this is not true, at least within the UK. This is to protect the health of the would-be mum and any babies conceived through treatment.

The average cost for a complete IVF cycle is currently around £5,000, not including medication, which on average can be between £2,000 - £3,000 depending on protocol. For US, 'according to the N.C.S.L., the average I.V.F. cycle can cost anywhere from $12,000 to $17,000 (not including medication). With medication, the cost can rise closer to $25,000.' (Fertility clinics abroad)

The following list from the Human Fertilisation and Embryology Authority (HFEA) demonstrates average success rates in the UK considering the age of the woman. Figures for US are according to Penn Medicine. Note that exact figures can vary slightly between individual clinics.

	UK	US
under 35	29%	above 20%
35-37	23%	17%
38-39	15%	11.1%
40-42	9%	5.7%
43-44	3%	2.3%
over 44	2%	0.6%

ICSI – This procedure is very similar to IVF except that instead of the egg and sperm being placed in a laboratory dish together, the sperm is injected into the egg to increase the chances of fertilisation.

The average cost of an ICSI cycle is currently around £500 - £1000 in the UK and $800 - $2,500 in the US on top of the IVF cost.

Paying for IUI/IVF/ICSI

There is funding available through the NHS in the United Kingdom for these procedures but, again, exact offers may vary. Most Clinical Commissioning Groups (CCGs) in each locality pay between 1-3 cycles. There are, however, restrictions on eligibility such as age, weight, smoking habits, and if the couple have a biological child already.

You can find out how many cycles your local CCG covers depending on where you live and what their eligibility criteria is. Due to discrepancies across the country, some individuals, and groups campaign for fairness on the number of cycles covered by the NHS. The difference between 1 and 3 cycles can mean a substantial difference in opportunities for a couple trying to conceive through this treatment.

Islamic ruling on IUI/IVF & ICSI

The Islamic ruling on the three mentioned treatments is that they are *halal* and within Islamic guidelines. Procedures for treatments involve medication usually injected in the female to manipulate and improve the natural job of hormones. The process of adding together the semen and eggs of the married couple is also a controlled method to what is naturally supposed to happen.

There are some arguments to suggest the act of masturbation required for collecting semen is *haram*. Whilst I am not a scholar, this does seem a stretch because the intent and purpose for the act in this scenario are entirely different from the act being done in the usual manner for the usual reasons away from fertility treatments.

In responding to the question 'Is it permissible to masturbate for the purpose of medical testing?', Al-Shaykh 'Abd Al-Al-Azeez ibn Humayd, said 'There is nothing wrong with that so long as there is a need for it' (Islamqa.info 2003).One other consideration to be mindful of is that a woman having the above treatments will have many internal scans as well as egg retrieval if and when needed. These scans or surgeries are carried out by male or female medical staff. As such, some Muslim women may worry about private parts or *awrah* being exposed but this is no different from scans and checks as well as labour experienced by any pregnant woman. These are required medical steps and I think there are little to no arguments that can be built on claiming it to be unacceptable in Islam.

Surgical Treatments

Surgical treatments are a huge benefit for many women and couples wanting to start a family. Surgical treatment options currently exist for both males and females depending on identified or suspected fertility issues.

For women, surgical treatments available in the UK include surgery to correct blocks in the fallopian tubes or to rectify health issues related to endometriosis. Some women have one or both fallopian tubes blocked, meaning that semen is restricted from traveling correctly to reach the eggs. The result is not being able to achieve pregnancy. The possibility of blocked tubes as well as the presence of endometriosis is checked during the early testing stages. Here is a list of common surgeries for females to help increase fertility. Detailed information can be found from the Human Fertilisation & Embryology Authority (HFEA), where much of the information on this section has been obtained.

* Keyhole surgery
* Hysteroscopic surgery
* Conventional surgery

For men, the main surgery option for fertility is called surgical sperm extraction, where sperm are surgically retrieved from the male. This is usually for men who have extremely low or no sperm. This can result from various things such as previous medical treatments, like chemotherapy, and/or other illnesses. There are 4 types of surgical sperm extractions obtainable in the UK which can be found on the HFEA website.

Islamic ruling on surgical treatments

All surgical treatments described above for both males and females are perfectly in line with Islamic guidelines in a similar way to other medical surgeries you may need at any time.

Egg Donor and Sperm Donor

Treatments involving egg or sperm donors are like IUI, IVF, and ICSI in terms of procedures, but with a big difference. When a couple opts for an egg or sperm donor or both, it means that someone else's egg or sperm outside of the marriage will be used. Therefore, a child conceived from this treatment will not be the biological child of either the mum (if the couple used an egg donor), the father (if they used a sperm donor), or either parent (if they used both egg and sperm donors).

Numerous people are willingly to donate eggs and sperm to fertility and medical clinics and remain anonymous. Other times people donate eggs or sperm to family members. For example, a sister or a close friend may donate her eggs to help a couple she knows and loves to have a child. Once a willing adult donates eggs or sperm, they no longer have legal rights to any children conceived from the donation.

Professional advice for a couple receiving egg or sperm donors is to use a registered clinic. This is so that appropriate screening and tests are carried out and legal papers drawn up to minimise confusion as to the parents of the child. Procedurally, IUI, IVF or ICSI treatments will follow an egg and/or sperm donor being chosen either through a clinic or through friends or family.

Egg and sperm donors in the UK are not allowed to be paid but a couple using this option may incur the below costs per cycle in *addition* to costs for IUI, IVF, or ICSI treatment. Prices vary hugely is the US for these options, but average costs according to Forbes Health for a full cycle using egg or sperm donor is given below:

	UK	US
Donor sperm	£35	$300-1,600
Donor egg	£700	(frozen) $14,000-$20,000
		(fresh) $27,000-47,000

Islamic ruling on Egg and Sperm Donation

The overwhelming evidence suggests that starting a family through egg or sperm donation is prohibited (*haram*) in Islam.

However, some reasons given are complicated. For some, the argument is about fornication, or *zina*. They argue that for a woman to fall pregnant from a man who is not her husband is *zina*, and thus a child from this union would be illegitimate. In the same way, they also argue that a man's sperm fertilising an egg from a woman that is not legally his wife is also *zina*.

Others feel an argument on *zina* in such cases is baseless. They claim that like with IVF, etc., sexual intercourse is not required to conceive a child. This is because eggs and sperm are collected separately and then put together in a laboratory dish, whether a couple is married or not.

Further problems with this option raised by many Muslims and people of knowledge are related to the issue of lineage. Islamically lineage (i.e., the bloodline of a person) is given utmost importance. Therefore, to conceive a child using donated eggs or sperm and then to carry the child and raise them as your own, where they may never know their biological parent(s), is incompatible with Islamic rulings on family and lineage.

Other social factors which make this option potentially non-viable for Muslim couples wanting to adhere to Islamic law is that children conceived through donors will often not know their biological parents and/or siblings. As rare as it may be, there is a possibility where children from the same donor but raised in different families could meet and marry without realising that they are biological siblings. This may cause extremely frightening ethical, social, and medical problems for those involved.

For example, a sperm donor in the UK can donate up to 10 families excluding their own. The outcome from this is a child conceived through a sperm donor in the UK could have blood siblings of up to 11 families across the country without knowing them.

European Council of Fatwa and Research said the following on a question about where a woman could use embryos developed through IVF with her husband yet frozen to be used later. In response, the scholars concluded '...But if she is separated from him through death, divorce or the like and thus is no longer under the bond of marriage with him, it will be unlawful to implant any of them and she should destroy them or what remains of them' (European Council of Fatwa and Research 1999). This response demonstrates that egg, sperm, or embryos from an unmarried couple are unlawful to use to create a child.

In conclusion, it's understood that 'all assisted reproductive technologies are permitted in Islam, if the semen source, ovum source, and the incubator (uterus) come from the legally married husband and wife during the span of their marriage' (Fadel HE 2007).

Surrogacy

Surrogacy refers to the situation where a couple finds a female outside of the relationship to carry a child for them. Procedure wise, the couple finds someone to be a surrogate for them privately or through a surrogate agency.

Once a surrogate is known to the couple personally or a match is made through an agency, IVF or ICSI will be used to develop embryos. The embryos will then be planted into the surrogate who will grow and carry the child to term and then deliver it.

Biologically, a child born through this method is the child of the couple and not the surrogate who carried the child. This is because the eggs are from the intended mother and sperm from the intended father (the couple). It's only after the embryo has been developed from the two parents that it's placed into the womb of the surrogate to house until birth.

There is also something called 'partial surrogacy' where the eggs and the womb of the surrogate are used along with the sperm of the male partner of the couple wanting a child.

A surrogate is normally used when there is a physical obstacle or difficulty in the intended mother carrying the child safely. It is also considered where there are recurrent miscarriages. Once pregnancy is complete, the surrogate delivers the baby naturally or via c-section, like any other pregnancy. Biological parents are usually present during labour, then the newborn is given to them upon birth.

Paperwork and agreements for all concerned parties involved are completed before pregnancy and/or during it. Having legal paperwork and contracts is essential for this method to protect all parties.

Surrogacy is smooth for many families and individuals, however, there are practical issues to consider. For example, in the UK, the recognised mother of a child conceived this way is often the woman who carried the child (the surrogate). When dealing with the matter of who a 'mother' is, Section 33(1) of the Human Fertilisation and Embryology Act 2008 states, 'The woman who is carrying or has carried a child as a result of the placing in her of an embryo or sperm and eggs, and no other woman is to be treated as the mother of the child' (legislation.gov.uk).

This means that in many cases the legally recognised mother is the one who carried and gave birth to the child (unless legal adoption has been completed) and therefore it is a tricky option that must be tread carefully.

In the UK, it is illegal for a surrogate to be paid; but couples using a surrogate do pay for expenses such as loss of earnings, travel costs, or extra medical bills until the baby is born and during a reasonable recovery period after birth. According to a report by Surrogacy UK, surrogates typically receive £10,000 - £15,000 in expenses. Costs for surrogacy in US is one of the highest in the world and can be as high as up to $200,000 in some states including medical and legal needs.

Islamic Ruling on Surrogacy

Before I began researching for this book, I automatically assumed surrogacy was *haram* and unacceptable in Islam.

In reality, I found a difference of opinion on this complicated and modern topic.

On the one side, there is a strong argument that says this method of conceiving a child is *haram* for multiple reasons. One of the reasons given is the idea of there being an element of *zina* and children from this method being illegitimate.

Additionally, issues of 'two mums' can occur as mentioned already. There have been cases in the UK and worldwide where the surrogate desires to keep the baby after birth, causing a struggle and usually a legal battle over who the rightful mother is.

Legislations in the UK on the matter previously referenced and the Islamic ruling on who a mother is share a similar view; as stated in the Quran 'their mothers are only those who gave birth to them' (Quran: 58:2). This *ayah* deals with the term '*waladna hum*' in Arabic which some suggest describes 'from conception to delivery'(Ilmgate.org) although this term simply put means to 'give birth', which could have never been without conception in the first place until recent medical techniques emerged. Therefore 'conception' is thus the rational deduction.

In surrogacy, the one who 'conceives' the child is the intended mother whose eggs are used but the one who 'gives birth' is the surrogate. Such points hammer home the spiritual and social complication for this treatment option.

The European Council of Fatwa and Research has also declared it 'impermissible for a woman to hire her womb to carry an embryo in it. It is impermissible even if it were done gratis, for this involves introducing the sperm of a man that is not her husband, and it would lead to mixing up and confusing ancestry or genealogy' (European Council of Fatwa and Research 2003).

Therefore, from an Islamic perspective, there are worrying entanglements to avoid that can cause harm on an individual as well as a societal level. Biologically, the child belongs to the woman whose eggs are used to conceive the child but the legal view in the UK and the Islamic view both suggest that the carrier, known as the surrogate, has a huge stake in the situation too. The surrogate mother and the baby coexist for nine months in a pretty much biological (and emotional) exchange, resulting in biological changes like breasts filling with milk in the surrogate mother, etc. and a strong bond in between. So, it is not only a matter of genealogy, but also psychological, too.

On the other side of the argument are those who say there is 'more goodness' than harm from such a situation. They make the point that since the embryo is developed scientifically (not naturally through intercourse) the placement of the embryo in the surrogate is not more than a transactional setup, leading to the womb of this surrogate being 'rented' as a 'host' to carry the child to full term with full understanding and agreement from all those involved.

They argue this transaction is acceptable as long as there is no compulsion and/or oppression against surrogates.

I referred to another form of surrogacy known as partial surrogacy where both the egg and womb of the surrogate are used. Islamically there is a clearer argument that this option is *haram* as it combines reservations on standard surrogacy coupled with the Islamic stance on egg donors.

As shown in this tiny bit of information, surrogacy is one of the most contentious and at times confusing options that may be open to a Muslim couple unable to carry their child. It has been included here in the hope of providing as much information as possible for you so that you can do your research to discover what is best for you as a couple, spiritually and practically.

Holistic Treatments

With regards to fertility, the term 'holistic treatments' refer to various options accessible to women or couples trying to conceive.

It may include any of the following:

1– Diet and exercise

This involves a focus on personal changes around diet and exercise. Many women who choose this route often spend time researching the effects of different foods on the body as well as looking into the needs of their own bodies. For example, there is ever-growing scientific research into the impact of the gut, often known as the 'second brain' on overall health, including fertility.

A quick google search can give you relevant talks, books, and articles on the gut indicating the state of the gut can and does massively impact overall health. For many people, many health problems such as headaches, skin issues, autoimmune disease, and infertility can be traced back to issues in the gut.

Thus, fixing or healing the gut can be an effective and healthy way to achieve optimum health. For many women and couples, it can restore and reverse health blocks that have thus far prevented a healthy pregnancy.

When going down this route, the exact plan or aim will differ greatly from one person to another. This depends on the current diet, current health complaints, and overall aim. For some, it could include cutting out caffeine, dairy, or meat.

Turning our attention to exercise; there is overwhelming evidence on the positive impact regular exercise can have on the body and mind. Furthermore, working out in a way that is personal and specific can aid pregnancy. For example, some women struggle with extra weight that can exacerbate existing health problems such as endometriosis or PCOS. This makes the need to exercise even more of a priority.

Other vital benefits can include positive effects on the brain, reduction of stress, and balancing hormones, all of which can improve the likelihood of achieving pregnancy depending on the situation and diagnosis.

If you feel this an option you want to explore, begin by doing some research then have a conversation with your doctor.

Thereafter you may wish to speak with a personal trainer and/ or a nutritionist or explore further information on diet and exercise from books, podcasts, and articles.

The main thing to be cautious about when looking into this is not to be overwhelmed. The amount of information on the topic is numerous and at times very conflicting. When I first decided to explore this as an option, I began by doing as much research as possible with a curious and critical eye.

The reality is every 'expert' will push their understanding of the topic. It can be challenging to ascertain the best approach for your body type or needs. Sometimes certain diets may do more harm and hence it is so important to check the credibility of the information provided. However, this can be life-changing for some, and with time and dedication you can learn a lot about food, exercise, and your body. It's good to find resources and people you trust to help you navigate it all.

A commitment to enhancing your health and fertility through holistic treatments and personal changes like diet and exercise can be expensive. It's important to be mindful that there is a certain level of investment in time and finance for this.

I urge anyone wanting to go down this route to dedicate and put some finance towards this goal regularly. The main cost here is food because a lot of diets for optimising health including fertility will require 'organic' foods and an increase in fresh fruit and vegetables. For those living in the UK and many western countries, buying organic food or ingredients you wouldn't use every day can cost a premium.

Additionally, while there are tons of free workout routines online and walking is also free and available to most of us around the world, some people will want the support, access, and accountability of a personal trainer and/or classes or local gyms, which will again cost money.

However, as advised to begin with, there is free information through the internet in many languages to get you started. The same goes for books as well.

2–Acupuncture

Acupuncture is a holistic treatment often recommended for better fertility. Medical experts don't agree on its effectiveness but there is a lot of information—although not all scientific—that does support the idea that acupuncture can improve fertility.

Acupuncture is the procedure of using small needles inserted into the face and body in specific areas depending on the health aim. The patient having acupuncture sits or lays down in a quiet place with the needles inserted for some time, usually between 30 to 60 minutes.

The needles are thought to increase and support blood flow and maintain balance in the body, including the hormones. It is historically part of Chinese medicine. There is something called Qi/Chi, which is very common in acupuncture and considered vital for improving overall health using this method. A simple online search or a discussion with an acupuncturist can provide more information on this.

Acupuncture is common and accessible in most parts of the world. In the UK it is extremely easy to find a local acupuncturist, especially if you live in one of the larger cities. A google search on 'acupuncturist near me' will flag up centres and individual practitioners close by.

Acupuncture is offered in both health centres specialising in holistic services as well as in personal homes or offices. Similar to other treatments, anyone wanting to use this treatment should take the time to research its suitability to their own needs. All practitioners in this field should be certified and experienced. It is possible to get a male or female practitioner depending on your need and preference, and a thorough check on the credibility and safety of the practitioner is a must.

It's important to be cautious that the environment used for acupuncture is clean and needles are used only once. Acupuncture is mainly painless and can be relaxing.

From a personal perspective, I have used acupuncture in the past and want to use it again in the future. Sadly, I didn't know enough to find a way to measure its effectiveness before, but I think I would try and find a way to do that when using it again in the future.

The cost for acupuncture can vary, but in the UK, it typically ranges between £50-100 per session. Some charities do group sessions for a fraction of the price, so this may be worth looking into.

3–Cupping/Hijama

Cupping, along with many other 'holistic' services, is a treatment frequently associated with Chinese medicine, but cupping, known as *hijama* in Arabic, is also an old Islamic tradition and a *sunnah*.

Cupping, or *hijama*, is done by placing 'cups' to specified areas on the body until these cups tighten and 'suck' in the skin, applying pressure on those areas.

The cups are left on those areas for a few minutes for suction to complete, then the practitioner removes the cups. In a process known as 'wet' cupping, the practitioner then cuts the area. This is not as painful as it sounds since the area has already been made numb from the suction.

The cutting releases blood which is understood to contain toxins that have been gathered from the body via the blood. The released blood is then discarded. 'Dry' cupping, where no cutting takes place, is also available mostly through Chinese medicine. Multiple cups are used in multiple spots in the body in one session of cupping. The expected outcome is improved overall health and it's an available treatment option to aid fertility naturally. Many people report many health benefits including improved energy.

Cupping is available in most parts of the world, including most cities and towns across the UK. With cupping, you also have the additional choice of using it in a Muslim setting or through other spaces that specialise in Chinese medicine.

Depending on your location, many Muslims, including myself, opt to have cupping done in a Muslim setting. For me, the additional spiritual element such as having Quran being recited or played in the background, the focus on '*sunnah* spots' or doing it on the 'white days' adds another dimension to the treatment.

When it comes to finding reliable scientific reports on the efficacy of cupping and/or acupuncture, there is nothing definitive.

However, there are countless anecdotal reports for both treatments related to fertility and non-fertility health. Many argue the placebo effect is the reason so many people feel cupping and/or acupuncture is beneficial to their health.

One case widely cited in platforms for health journals such as The National Centre of Biotechnology Information (NCBI) shares the story of a 28-year-old Mexican woman who successfully conceived following 28 sessions of acupuncture accompanied by cupping therapy without other medical interference.

Many Muslims already trust and use cupping because of the position it has in Islam and prophetic medicine. For example, the Prophet (PBUH) said 'The best medicine with which you treat yourselves is *hijama*' (Sahih Al Bukhari Hadith No. 537).

Also, Abu Hurairah (RA) reported the Messenger (PBUH) said 'Whoever performs cupping (*hijama*) on 17th, 19th and 21st of the lunar month, then it is a cure for every disease' (Sunan Abu Dawud Hadith No. 3861).

Still, with all holistic or alternative treatments, caution is advised. If cupping is something you are considering, it is paramount you use someone trained, who performs these services in a sterile and clean environment. Too many people access this treatment inside people's homes.

Even though receiving these services in groups is common, it can still be dangerous. The level of sterilising, the means of disposing the blood, and training level of the practitioners are all questionable.

If you can find a trustworthy, professional, and clinical environment, then I highly recommend using that as an alternative to informal sessions in people's homes. Of course, there are independent and highly trained practitioners delivering this service in their home or personal office, but due diligence on your part is highly advised.

Other people are confident in cupping themselves. Only you can decide if you feel you have the skills and knowledge to do this treatment on your own in a safe way. However, often specific points you might want to do, including those thought to be *sunnah* spots, are located on the back of the body. Therefore, being able to fully complete cupping treatment on your own may prove challenging.

There is a wide range to the cost of cupping, but you can expect anything between £30 to £60 per session in the UK and $40 to $80 per session in America.

4–Herbal Medicine

Herbal medicine in this situation refers to a mixture of various herbs that are consumed as food or drink. The main ingredients usually involve lots of plants. The appeal for this by many is the natural aspect of it.

There are a multitude of plants that are suggested to have medicinal or healing powers. The form in which various herbs are offered include teas, drops taken orally or topically, tablets, powders, and more.

It is irresponsible for me to list here any herbs commonly associated with boosting fertility as many have zero to little credibility. Also, some may have negative side effects. The only one I will suggest here is the black seed or black cumin. Black seed exists in several forms from seeds to powder to liquid.

The reason I have chosen to highlight black seed as opposed to some of the others is that it has been celebrated as an extremely powerful herbal medicine within prophetic medicine. Abu Huraira narrated: 'I heard the apostle saying, "There is healing in black cumin for all diseases except death"' (Sahih Al Bukhari Hadith No. 5688).

Herbal treatments are sold in a variety of ways. They are sold online, in herbal or health stores, made at home, or purchased from individuals selling them independently.

Although natural and herbal treatments can aid general health, and in some cases fertility, it is crucial that anyone wanting to try this method for improving fertility health is careful about what they consume and from whom. Extra care and research are needed for ingredients in all herbal products and any apparent scientific research for its health claims.

The cost of herbal medicine is extremely wide-ranging. It depends on the product and where the product is purchased. Financially you will want to plan for extra costs if herbal medicine is something you want to consider alongside or as an alternative to mainstream medical treatments.

Some herbs can be very costly, so you want to be extra sure that anything you decide to buy, and use is cost-effective and can aid health.

5–Taking Supplements

Supplements in this context refers to adding various dietary supplements to increase or improve vitamins already created within the body. There are often a multitude of negative consequences if you lack some key vitamins.

For women and couples looking to improve or heal fertility problems, this is another angle for consideration when looking at holistic or alternative medicine. Forms in which supplements are ingested or topically applied vary in a similar way to herbal medicine. Depending on personal aims and preferences as well as the required vitamin, you can use supplements as tablets, powders, injections, or spray on.

In the UK and in most countries, you can get basic blood tests if you suspect that you are deficient in important vitamins. Initial tests following a conversation with your GP about fertility will likely mean you go through numerous testing to check your specific vitamin levels.

The GP or consultant will focus on key vitamins but there is a possibility that many others will not be analysed during preliminary tests; it is worth knowing which are overlooked. You can get tested privately for most vitamins or those that are not routinely available in the NHS if you prefer.

A large range of vitamins are sold in supermarkets, pharmacies, health stores, and/or online in many countries. If you think you may need vitamin supplements, know that further research on most points made in this section will be necessary.

It's important for us to know our bodies as much as possible and to question why we would need extra vitamins in addition to a 'good' diet. The food we eat and the way it interacts with our body is the biggest role in vitamin optimisation. Remember that even natural vitamins can be detrimental to your health and well-being if ingested in improper amounts.

Whilst I emphasise that I am not a doctor or a health expert, some of the most important, basic and largely agreed upon vitamins needed for optimum health, and by extension fertility, include folic acid, magnesium, vitamin D, iron, and coenzyme Q10.

It's easy to trust and invest a lot of time, energy, and money into consuming more and more vitamins with the best intentions but receive little positive impact. Furthermore, there are people everywhere able and willing to exploit the desperation of so many women and couples desiring a child. Most holistic treatments don't have huge amounts of rigorous and scientific research backing their health claims. Additionally, unlike treatments such as IVF, there is little regulation in this field in most countries. It is paramount that you heavily scrutinise holistic or alternative services and products claiming health benefits, especially concerning fertility, and that you acquire information from credible sources.

6–Ruqyah/exorcism

Ruqyah can be translated in English as exorcism, which can be confusing for many people of all faiths. *Ruqyah*, in its simplest form, is someone having passages of the Quran recited on them for healing. In many cases, it is carried out by someone considered to be proficient in the Quran.

This person may be a sheikh or at least able to recite and ideally have a good grasp of the meaning of each *ayah* recited. The Quran is recited with the aim of it being a cure for an individual or group of people. Many people maintain it's more favourable to perform *ruqyah* on oneself instead of having it recited by others.

In Islam, it's widely believed that beings called 'jinns', made from smokeless fire (where humans are made from clay and angels from light) exist. The purpose of their creation is the same as humans: 'I did not create jinn and mankind except that they worship me' (Al-Quran: 51:56).

Like humans, there are both benevolent and evil jinns. The evil jinns can cause harm to humans, namely by possessing them. This possession can cause an individual to suffer physically, mentally, and spiritually. *Ruqyah* for treatment is the main cure to banish or exorcise a jinn from one's life and/or body.

Additionally, *ruqyah* can be used to counteract harm caused by evil eye and black magic, both of which can affect one's health, wealth, or relationships.

Ruqyah is a unique and spiritually based alternative treatment open to Muslims. It can be used for improving general health or as a form of treatment for specific health concerns, including fertility.

Ruqyah is available in most parts of the world. It's accessed either by finding someone online or by word of mouth through your local Muslim community.

It's particularly important to iterate here that all listed 'holistic treatments' are to be explored with extreme caution and none more so than *ruqyah*.

Extreme caution is necessary because dealing with *ruqyah* and its connected elements is essentially part of the 'unseen world'. The difficulty in this is that similar to with herbal medicine, there is no shortage of deceitful people who will exploit others in their vulnerability, their need, and their lack of knowledge in certain areas.

The abuse of trust and power in using *ruqyah* is widespread in the Muslim community across the world. Many so-called *raqi*s will charge people extensive amounts of money to promise a cure from evil eye, jinn possession, and most commonly, black magic.

What makes it so dangerous is so many Muslims trust the so-called *raqi*s hastily. These *raqi*s market themselves as sincere and knowledgeable in this field as well as the *deen*.

Many think there's no harm in someone reciting the Quran but there is a great deal of potential harm because the level of deceit these people employ and exploit in these situations is immense.

A lot of people use this as their main vehicle of abusing power, increasing their wealth and self-importance.

It is also possible to perform *ruqyah* oneself or by a loved one. There is some evidence Islamically that support the idea that this is the most encouraged and preferred way to do it.

Ruqyah can get very costly, and hence why it is so highly exploited. In the UK, a *ruqyah* session can cost between £50 to £150 on average but some packages can cost tens of thousands.

***

With all the treatments listed, it is important to manage your expectations. For most people, there isn't an 'easy fix'. Pregnancy, motherhood, or a cure from ailments may occur as a combination of treatments and time. Other times, as we know, things happen when they are supposed to happen, regardless of treatment.

I encourage you to have a balance in being hopeful for success with treatments and an understanding that it may not have the exact outcome you desire.

There is a big responsibility on your shoulders when it comes to understanding and accessing suitable treatments for your personal needs, as there is the same responsibility on my shoulders for my needs.

It requires each of us to go that extra mile to research, question, test, and keep learning. No one else can do this for you. It can get overwhelming, but without the due diligence of research and knowledge, you can easily get sucked into a 'miracle cure' that turns out to be fake or harmful.

While mainstream medical treatments such as IVF are not perfect or free from exploitation, those administering and managing them are generally professionals sworn to save life, protect people, and avoid causing harm. This industry is also heavily regulated, which is NOT the case for alternative medicines or treatments.

Treatments Abroad

The final possibility in the list of options for Muslim women and couples is to use treatments abroad. Reasons for choosing treatments abroad can include more affordable treatment options, higher outcomes of success or wanting to work with a specific clinic or consultant.

In a similar way to every treatment described in this part of the book, thorough research is crucial before using any treatments abroad. Possibility of complications, language barriers, and setbacks such as different laws and regulations for treatments, may result in negative or unwanted outcomes and stress.

Furthermore, a key consideration is the cost. This is extremely difficult to predict because there is so much to consider, such as country of choice, treatment required, travel and accommodations. Besides, treatments such as IVF can be stressful and time-consuming in the best of times, so having to travel to another country for egg retrieval and other appointments can cause a further burden for some.

Proactivity with caution throughout the TTC journey is vital. This is no exception. Over the years, I have witnessed trends for certain countries that become a 'hotspot' for accessing fertility treatments sometimes for no clear reason at all.

I caution against this approach to avoid unnecessary stress, confusion, or harm. Making decisions and approaching treatments with a personalised and highly researched manner is always advisable.

In conclusion to this section, the leading message I want to impart on you is that you must take ownership of this journey. It's tempting to either do nothing or hand over the journey and decisions to 'experts'. But with the best of intentions by medical staff and others, no one will ever care about your health or happiness as much as you.

It's incumbent on you to find the strength to own the steps required for the task. It's your job to ask questions, compare data, look for alternatives, manage timing and so much more. Through the role of managing and influencing these important steps, you can increase the chances of achieving your desired goals in the most suitable way possible.

My new approach to accessing and receiving treatments

One reason I implore you to own and understand this challenge is that for the longest time I did the opposite. You may already be ahead of me in this regard, and if so, I admire your tenaciousness.

In my experience of treatments in trying to conceive, whilst I was proactive in pursuing treatment quickly, I was never knowledgeable about procedures or other details. I did what I was told when I was told.

It is sad for me to inform you that I only began trudging through old notes on my previous tests and treatments in the past year. It's only during this time that I have begun to understand it all a bit better. I want to blame the science and medical jargon that is especially difficult to decipher, but to be brutally honest, I was the same regarding holistic treatments.

I felt it was not my place to be an 'expert' in my body, my treatments, my situation. Whilst I know my approach served me well then, I do think my belief overall to 'leave it others' was a mistaken belief, and I aim to do differently this time around to exemplify myself and live the message I harp on about. To own and be proactive in all aspects of this brutal battle.

In a previous chapter, I explained how my husband and I took a 4-and-a-half-year hiatus from the gruelling world of TTC through treatments but had planned to embark on it again soon.

As I write this, all plans to throw ourselves into it have been postponed as the world has been gripped for almost a year thus far by a sudden and frightening virus called coronavirus (Covid-19). Nevertheless, exhausting every avenue to become parents remains a priority and the focal point of all our goals.

My approach this time will be the absolute opposite to the woman I described above who went through the steps for treatments such as IVF but knew or understood very little about them.

I am giving myself a crash course in understanding holistic or alternative treatments as well, including the ones listed. I aim for us to use alternative methods to improve overall health before and alongside using mainstream medical treatments again.

I do believe that a suitable diet, exercise, acupuncture, cupping, etc. will add value and positive impact on the journey, as will counselling. My aim with it all is for me to be as physically, mentally, and emotionally strong as possible, before immersing myself in that world again. Additionally, I want to understand every protocol and procedure once I do undergo treatment.

To be honest and transparent, this had been a big concern for me. I worried it would all be too overwhelming. A huge criterion that allowed me to love life and enjoy it fully during the previous years of checks and treatments was not allowing myself to be sucked into it all so drastically.

I actively avoided my life revolving around treatments and pregnancy tests, but I feel now is the perfect time for me to go all in. I feel more equipped to find a balance in using the tools and information I have at my disposal, including much of what I have shared throughout this book. I hope you too can also use these tools and information to help you navigate it all in a safe way as well.

A structured and tangible way to possibly achieve this balance whilst being engrossed in research (if that is where you currently are), is to allocate a specific time for research for both mainstream and alternative treatments and anything else you need to learn about in TTC.

For example, one day a week could be dedicated to this activity alongside working on fun or important personal projects and goals. For example, spare 3-5 hours one day a week and do not work on it outside of that time frame.

Additionally, keep an eye on all the other parts of the 'Wheel of Life' as shown in Chapter 1, and ask yourself the following questions:
* Am I spending time seeing friends and family whose company I enjoy?
* Are my husband and I spending quality time together not related to TTC? Are we creating happy memories?
* Am I looking after my physical, emotional and mental health?
* Or am I allowing the task of becoming a mum to consume my every move?

What next?

A key take-away from part 2 is for you to be encouraged to take action. To benefit from the information provided, it's important to choose to act as soon as possible to achieve your desire of having your child(ren).

As Muslims, we accept that *dua* (supplication) is powerful and truly a weapon to survive life, but we also know, we must live by the understanding that we are responsible for putting in the effort.

We must play our part; sitting back and praying about it whilst not moving forward nor striving for change is unlikely to yield the fruits we desire.

This message is especially for you; if you have yet to explore treatment options in any meaningful way, such as having tests, going through treatment, etc. Those that want to take action but are held back by finance, for example, will still need to play their part such as exploring what is possible and raising money for their chosen treatment.

As you move forward in your action plan, ask yourself:

1.What treatment do we want to explore next, whether it is a repeat (another round of IVF, for example) or something new?

2.What finance or time will we need to invest in this part of the journey?

3.What else can I try or research further to increase my chances of motherhood/parenthood?

PART 3

YOUR FAMILY, YOUR OPTIONS

Your Family, Your Options

This section of the book will help you to explore creating, designing, and working for a family that is right for you.

Almost every woman I have had the pleasure to chat with or heard talk about infertility has said the same thing irrespective of faith or ethnic background: Each one has expressed shock at where she has found herself. Shocked by this unpredicted hurdle in her life.

There is a genuine and understandable challenge in dealing with the loss of the expectation of becoming parents when they had desired.

They find themselves swimming against the tide of trying to conceive for a year, 5 years, 15 years, or more. There is a loss to overcome. Heartache to endure. Information to digest, and so much more.

I want to assure you (and myself) that there is a world of options out there that allows us to seek a new dream, a new picture, and a new format of what our family can look like.

Each one of these options has its pros and cons like all things in life. Furthermore, they all go against the grain in some way, and they are certainly unlikely to be what you dreamt of for motherhood before you had to face the monster that is infertility. However, each choice has its beauty and blessings.

Every option will require thinking outside the box, putting to rest the idea you once held about what your family would be. It will require strength and independent thinking and action to carve out your happiness. To be bold and go for what you want especially regarding options that may be seen as odd or strange.

Note that regardless of cultural biases, each option presented is permissible within Islam.

Option 1: Lasting marriage and a child-free life

The first option available to you and your spouse is the decision to remain married to each other and live out the rest of your life child-free or until Allah gifts you children. We must assume that a couple desperate for children may only ever reach this point once they've exhausted all TTC possibilities.

There is an essence of this being 'unnatural' and unsettling because it goes against the 'norm'. It goes against expectations of marriage. It is not what we dreamt about but let's be honest, none of this was part of the dream. None of it was part of the expectation. For example, IVF injections, years of heartbreak and confusion were never part of our plan, wherever this journey ends.

The situation in which you and I now find ourselves forces us to think differently. To decide on a new 'normal' whatever that looks like for us.

Therefore, it is healthiest and most constructive for us to come to terms with that. It may take a minute. We may need to do our own rituals, or duas to overcome and let go of the expectations.

This doesn't mean we lose hope of carrying and raising our biological children if we are still in the midst of this journey, and particularly if we are in the early days or have not yet tried everything in our power. What it does mean, though, is that we will let go of what we thought our life would be and make decisions based on what it actually is.

The option, therefore, to remain married, to be committed, to make each other a priority, and to forge a life that is full of joy, wisdom and freedom is highly possible and not a decision to judge negatively.

Are you struggling with this concept because, in your mind, getting married meant having a baby too? This thought process can be changed and as discussed in the chapter on marriage, your marriage should always be separate and sacred, independent of children.

By choosing this option, the world opens differently for you. Diverse opportunities to have an impact, to leave a legacy, and to fulfil your purpose are attainable. Your life can be one with meaning.

This is better suited for couples who can come to terms with it being just the two of them. Exhausting TTC options, having discussions, seeking counselling, etc. may come before a couple decides on this option, that they can be happy and content in their small family of two. This may not be so suitable for couples where one or both feel they must raise children in some capacity to have a meaningful life. You have to believe in and understand your decision.

Social pressure—a theme that appears in almost every corner of this journey—is a major concern for couples considering this option. Family, friends, and the community at large may not understand this choice and may encourage the couple to separate if they are unable to have children.

This social pressure for a couple to separate is heightened if a medical reason has been identified with either the male or female but more so if it's thought to be with the women. This is heart-breaking and placing unnecessary pain on a couple already battling with infertility.

One way to cope with this pressure is to make your decision and the marriage itself as solid as possible privately. Therefore, negative comments and suggestions will have minimal negative impact on your peace of mind. Sincere, recurring conversations between you and your husband are important for you to help each other through it.

It may be that either one or both of you change your mind about the decision at some point; this is always more manageable through honest communication. To begin to embark on a decision such as this, an understanding of why this is the right decision for you both is non-negotiable. Having that conviction and clarity will anchor you during the harder times and keep you grounded when emotions spiral out of control.

Option 2: Adoption

Adoption is the means of legally becoming the parent of a child that is not biologically yours. Private and informal adoptions also exist, but these provide much less security than formal adoption.

Within the Muslim community, there are many misunderstandings about adoption and its permissibility, with a tremendously high number of Muslims believing that adoption is impermissible in Islam. However, not only is adoption allowed in Islam, but it is also encouraged. Adoption is a *sunnah* and is considered a form of worship.

Shortly we will discuss the matter of adoption in Islam in more detail, but first, let's look more closely at the personal benefits of adoption and how one goes about it.

Let's begin now with the question: Why adopt? For a great number of people, the simple answer is because they want to be a parent. It's less about having a biological child and more about the reality of being a parent.

To them, it means having children to love, mould, protect, and raise so that those children can thrive and have fulfilling lives. It is an option that meets the need to be a parent and enjoy full family life.

Additionally, this option provides couples—whether they have biological children or not—the opportunity to give adopted children the love and security they may not have otherwise had.

Most children needing adoption are in or will go into state care or orphanages. They don't have permanent adults in their lives to take care of them. Thus, adoption is the best opportunity to give such children a brighter and better future.

Several agencies around the world specialise in formal adoption. The rules and procedures will differ from country to country, so the guidelines used as a basis for information in this part will refer to the laws and rules of adoption in the UK.

Domestic adoption in the United States can be a difficult process but can be arranged through local states, adoption agencies and or independently.

Domestic adoption within the UK is through local authorities, also known as councils or adoption agencies. UK citizens and residents can get relevant information from their local council's website. Couples or single people interested in adoption will have the opportunity to attend meetings and information sessions within local authorities and or agencies.

Furthermore, relevant information on adoption and its rules are available on individual council websites, but the gov.uk website is a good starting point to gather initial information.

Who can adopt?

Most adults over the age of 21 can apply to become adoptive parents regardless of faith and/or background or relationship status. You need to be over 21 years of age but there is no upper age limit. Broadly speaking, the only criteria to automatically rule someone out in the UK is them or a family member having a criminal conviction or caution related to children or serious sexual offenses (Adoption UK). One other important requirement is that the child must be able to have their own bedroom, whether you own or rent the property. Each application is dealt with case by case, but it's important to note that it is a lengthy process.

If this is something you want to consider then contacting your local authority or attending an open information session is a great place to begin.

Adoption in Islam

Adoption in Islam is as old as Islam itself and highly encouraged. The Prophet SAW himself had an adopted son, Zayd ibn Harithah. A further look into this practice makes it clear that it was highly encouraged by the early Muslims.

A great number of prominent Muslims over the centuries, including many that were proficient in the Quran, the founders of all 5 *madhab*s (e.g., Hanafi, Shafi'i, etc.), as well as numerous hadith collectors, were either adopted themselves or had adopted and raised children that were not biologically their own.

This is discussed in much more detail in an excellent series of lectures compiled in 2017 by sheikh Omar Suleiman exploring Adoption and Fostering in Islam, and in particular a deep look at the *fiqh* of Adoption and Fostering in Islam. This video series is available on YouTube on the Yaqeen Institute channel.

This material delves deep into the virtues, *fiqh*, and reward of adopting and or fostering in Islam. Even a limited look into this topic of adoption and Islam quickly demonstrates this is a highly recommended action rather than something prohibited. The Yaqeen Institute's video series mentioned above and other lectures, articles, and/or books that cover the topic demonstrate this easily with plenty of evidence directly from the teachings of Islam.

Young children and babies needing to be adopted are usually orphans because one or both parents have passed. Other reasons leading to a child being in the care of the state is because one or both parents are alive but are unable to look after the child due to ill health, such as mental illness or substance abuse.

The job of stepping up to raise, love, and protect children that are in need in this way is a duty and a great opportunity from a spiritual perspective. The vast majority of Muslims across the globe are very familiar with the famous saying of the Prophet (SAW), "I and the person who looks after an orphan and provides for him, will be in Paradise like this," putting his index and middle fingers together (Sahih Al-Bukhari Hadith No. 6005).

This is a hadith that many of us often think about when raising funds for charities that look after children. Although my intention is not to undermine the great reward and duty of looking after orphans financially, we also need to look after them by providing them with a family, home, education, and security.

- What if adoption was not so scary?
- What if adoption was what was meant for you all this time?
- Is there a world where you can allow yourself to contemplate the possibility that adoption is for you and part of your perfectly planned destiny?

My aim is not to influence you, but rather to encourage you

to see it as an option to explore. There is a gift and an opportunity in this for the right Muslim couple who wish to give that love and security to an orphan child.

This opportunity that I describe as a possible gift provides a huge level of personal gain for an adoptive parent as it meets the desire to be a parent as well as provides significant spiritual benefits. In Islam, all 'good' acts are an act of worship depending on the intention. This includes ordinary activities or life events such as work, studying, exercise, getting married, and parenting. Thus, there is the opportunity for an enhanced level of reward for the one who steps up to adopt and start a family or add to it in this way.

For many Muslims, the issue of *mahram* once the adoptive child becomes of age is a concern. Fortunately, there are several practical ways that this can be overcome.

For example, an adoptive mother can breastfeed an adoptive child; once the child is breastfed in this way, that child becomes *mahram* for her, for her husband and any offspring they have naturally. 'Under Islamic Sharia law, breastfeeding an infant three to five or more feeds when the child is under two years gives the adopted child the rights of a birth child' (La Leche League International 2015).

There are detailed *fiqh* rules to consider this but to keep it basic for our purposes, here are some essential notes.

A woman who has recently adopted a baby or is about to adopt one can speak with her GP about accessing medication to help with lactation. This is possible for many women even without ever being pregnant or giving birth. The medications that make this possible are usually designed to increase breast milk for new mums. A well-known and common pill which is often prescribed is called domperidone.

This drug is considered safe, especially for short-term use, and is intended to trigger lactation. It is available on prescription once approved by a doctor.

Since breastfeeding is highly respected and encouraged in Islam, a 'wet nurse'—a woman who breastfeeds a child that is not biologically hers—was widely used amongst Muslims, usually when the biological mother was unable to breastfeed. This is still common in some parts of the world and new breast milk 'banks' are opening up across certain cities in the West at least.

Prophet Muhammad SAW himself had wet nurses as an infant. The common practice for this among the early Muslims means that a woman is permitted to breastfeed an infant whom she did not birth. Combined with modern technology and medicine, it now means that an adoptive mother can explore this route to create that bond and overcome *mahram* issues, which many Muslim households worry about.

The Holy Quran clearly states, 'Let another woman suckle (the child) on the (mother's) behalf' (65:6), and 'Forbidden to you are ... your mothers that have suckled you and your foster-sisters' (23:4).

Beyond the *mahram* issue, another concern about adoption from an Islamic perspective is the issue of inheritance.

The concern stems from Quranic verses dealing with inheritance that refer to '*awladakum*' (your children) (Quran 4:11), which clearly discusses blood children. Whilst that is a legitimate query and a clear ruling within the *deen*, other parts of the Quran inform us to write a will for the '*aqrabeen*' (close ones) (Quran: 2:83). This negates the problem of inheritance; clearly the Quran encourages us to leave a will for those that are the 'close ones' which can include other family members, like adopted children, who are not mentioned.

Furthermore, there is so much to give an adopted child whilst you are alive, allowing them to benefit and thrive from your parenting. All this provision, care, and love are added to your good deeds, as well as knowing you did right by your child.

The third important issue to be aware of is the issue of whether the family name of the child can be changed. At the onset, we need to remember that family lineage is very important in Islam. Family that forms around a lawfully married couple is considered necessary for healthy generations and social order. Thus, in an ideal Muslim society, blood relations are recognised and honoured. Everyone, including an adopted child, has the right to know his or her biological ancestors, and they should be told about this at an appropriate age while making sure they continue to feel safe and not alienated. 'Family name' sometimes comes in the middle of this challenge between preserving blood lineage and the child being fully embraced by the new adopted family. Can the adopting family give their surname to the child? What does Islam say about this?

Again, this is not a book on Islamic *fiqh*, so you need to do your own research about this. But it may be helpful to note here the distinction between different systems of naming. While patronymic is the name derived from one's biological father, the modern surname system does not necessarily refer to biological inheritance. Surname can be likened to *nisba*, an attribution indicating one's affiliation to a place or tribe. While there is a general knowledge that the adopted child's surname cannot be changed, this distinction is clearing the way: as long as the child's patronymic is preserved, maybe like a middle name, and on the birth certificate and other official records, the surname of the adopting family can be taken in the sense of *nisba*. Besides, taking the family name of another person has been allowed in Islam not only in cases of adoption, but also for various reasons like companionship, as a sign of alliance, staying long with them, or having studied with them.

What is forbidden in Islam is to give the "full name" of the adopting father which suggests the child is his own – such a claim has legal consequences in terms of inheritance as well as affecting the rules of modesty inside home.

As previously discussed, the topic of lineage is highly protected in Islam and the family name of that child must be maintained throughout his or her life. If the name is unknown, then there are other options, but simply listing the child under the patronymic of the adopted father is not permitted.

Learning this often comes as a shock to many people since secular laws, especially in the West, are quite different from Islam in this regard, and when people are not aware of different naming systems. In the UK and most Western cultures (as well as many non-Western cultures) it's acceptable for women to change their last name to that of their husbands, so that the entire nuclear family carries the same last name. Similarly, an adoptive child would be given that name too.

For some people, it can take a moment to come to terms with this situation, especially when they don't know the difference between a surname (which can be changed in the *nisba* sense) and a patronymic (which should be preserved with the biological lineage).

In the grand scheme of things, this is only as big of a deal as one wants to make it. Many countries have adopted different norms and rules in this matter, so the situation varies from nation to nation. As Muslim women, we don't have the same surnames as our children in most cases anyway, birth or adopted, so this makes very little difference in that regard. For the father, I also think this can easily be managed; an adopted child keeping his surname only sounds strange or abnormal in comparison to Western or Christian cultures. The truth is that the Islamic view on this makes a lot of sense whilst making very little difference in the everyday life between the child and parent. Assuming that many readers of this book will be Muslims living in the West, it is likely that eventually they may have to deal with the surname situation. Given this context, they have to be aware of the psychological consequences their decision might have for the child and for themselves at home, at school, and among the larger family.

A couple of years ago I sat in a café with a lovely young Muslim woman who had been TTC for almost 10 years at the time. We talked about options, and adoption came up, as it inevitably does. In discussing practical considerations, such as the family name, I remember how the young woman was rather startled by the idea that a child she and her husband adopt would not have the husband's name. Her emotional stance on it was that it seemed harsh and she would for sure change her child's surname if she were to adopt so that said child would 'feel' part of the family.

I understood her sentiments. And she is not alone in having these feelings. Yet, as noted above, the difference a name makes is only as important as we make it. Secondly, giving the adopting family's surname (in the *nisba* sense) to the child is not disallowed as long as – again as explained above – the child's patronymic name is also preserved. This looks like a sound Islamic option for Muslim families searching for a legal ruling. In the Fiqh of Adoption and Fostering in Islam series previously mentioned, Sh Omar Suleiman states '...*it's ok for the last name of a person to be changed as long as the lineage is preserved in some other way*". He goes on the explain the permissibility of changing the last name of an adopted child if their original family name is included as a 'middle name' or hyphenated but shouldn't be eradicated altogether.

But, to reiterate, this is not a *fiqh* book. Every family might have unique cultural and legal circumstances; so, I encourage everyone to do their own research and seek consultancy from scholars and experts in this matter. Like anything else in life, our purpose as Muslims is to worship Allah (SWT) as He guided us to; therefore, breaking His rules to satisfy our desires in any situation may prove problematic for us in the long term.

The safeguarding of lineage is extremely important and can also allow adoptees to know a bit more about who their biological parents were and where they came from. This can be a gift for an adoptee rather than it being something negative. In some instances, a name change is encouraged for safety reasons and cases have to be considered case by case.

Different countries have different laws regarding adoption in many ways, including name change, so it is paramount that you do a thorough investigation suitable for your location.

In the UK and I suspect in other parts of the world—there are varied routes to adopting. One route into adoption is to adopt internationally. You can work with relevant agencies to be matched with a child in another part of the world. For some, this can allow adopting a child from their birth country or family's country of origin. Alternatively, the route to adoption can also be completed domestically within the country of residence. Formal adoption (through local authorities and agencies) and informal adoption (through people the couple already knows) are both possible.

Whether adoption is international, domestic, via agencies or through people you know, the legal side of adoption is vital. All necessary paperwork, checks, and agreements must be completed at each stage and ideally through a professional legal team. This is to protect all parties involved including the adopted child(ren) and adoptive parents.

Where is the love?

One issue potential adoptive parent commonly consider is the issue of love. A few questions that often arise include: Will I be able to love my adoptive child as I would have loved my biological child? Will my family and community accept my adoptive child(ren)?

Whilst these are natural questions, it is important to invest the necessary time and emotional effort to work through them thoroughly. For example, the first question is one that you and your spouse have control over, and whilst I think it is a common concern, many people who adopt do have an abundance of love to give.

They long to be called Mum and Dad and want to enjoy the ups and downs of raising little humans. They have enough love to pour to any child they adopt. However, your views on love and adoption have so much to do with yourself, your character, your upbringing, and your views of the world. Thus, after some examination and honest analysis of yourself and your situation you should be able to answer this and similar questions for yourself.

The question about acceptance of your adopted child by your wider circle is slightly out of your control. You cannot force extended family members, friends, or community to accept your newly built family.

You have to consider how much weight their reaction holds for you. How will their potential non-acceptance of your adoptive child affect you? Is there room for change or growth from them once the child is in your life? More importantly, does any of it put the child in danger if those people fail to accept and embrace them?

This is again something you can work through as a couple in a way that is relevant to your situation. It does require bravery, independent thinking, and a certain level of certainty about the desire to adopt before any child is placed with you.

The process for adoption is an understandably rigorous one. It often entails trained social workers and other relevant professionals assessing applications with numerous stages including health tests, accommodation assessments, and interviews with family and friends.

Option 3: Fostering

Fostering refers to the temporary care for a child or children for as little as one night or as long as many years. The process is usually less rigorous and permanent than adopting but it can be suitable for some couples who want to be parents in some capacity.

In the UK, adults aged 21 and over can apply to become a foster carer. There is less choice and less control through this route of taking care of a child. For example, you have less choice in which child is given to you. You also have less control over the length of time that a child is placed with you. They can be taken back at any point when either their parent, another suitable family member, adoptive parents, or another foster family is found.

This is not suitable for everyone but it's something that may be explored to allow someone the opportunity to help raise a child, even for a short time. It is an opportunity to love and be loved by a child. Many foster placements last for many years.

However, this is also very tricky for some emotionally, as having to 'give back' children in your foster care after bonds have been made is heart-breaking and beyond what many people can cope with. It might also be a sensitive issue for those unable to conceive yet or those who have experienced miscarriages. Having to let go of children after forming special relationships may prove to be too difficult.

Additionally, individuals like myself who have experienced loss—loss of a parent, loss of being a parent, loss of a country, or loss of a friend—need to assess their suitability and their ability to add value to being a foster parent.

A positive outcome from fostering is that for some people, it becomes a steppingstone to adopting. For example, if you yourself have reservations about adopting or you're worried about the reaction of extended family members, fostering may be a way to allow yourself and others to see what your family could be. To see your family set up change and be different from the 'norm' could be life changing. Furthermore, in time you could adopt a child or children whom you have been fostering.

The experience of fostering can reduce this lifestyle or family set-up being seen as drastic or abnormal and allows you to get used to potentially adopting. However, this should not be the main reason you foster as there are no guarantees that fostering will automatically lead to adoption.

Unlike adoption, fostering, which is designed to be temporary, is paid by local authorities. In the UK, a foster parent has paid wages which take into account their personal time and skills used to help raise the child. They are also given an allowance to help cover food, clothes, medical bills and education for the child.

Again, within the UK, initial steps into fostering usually involve completing a brief online form to indicate interest. This is followed by a telephone call from your local authority who will give you information for the next steps, including being invited to an information session, meeting, or completing further application forms.

There are substantial differences in procedures, protocols, and legal obligations regarding most, if not all, of the options covered in this book depending on your geographic location. Hence, although you may use the information presented as a general guideline which may provide some awareness or raise some needed questions, it is crucial that you conduct further research relevant to your location and personal circumstance.

Option 4: Polygyny/Polygamy

Polygyny is when a man has more than one wife.

Unlike other aspects of this book, the following option may be uncomfortable for some and highly offend others. The inclusion of this topic, especially in a book that is clearly for women can make certain people feel betrayed or let down and or that it's unnecessary.

However, I strongly believe that this is a needed discussion, and it would be unjust for the message of this book to leave it out. With that in mind, it's important to note that many Muslims don't fully agree with the practice of polygyny in the 21st century for various reasons. Even with that taken into consideration, this is an issue that many Muslim couples struggling to have children will talk about, be thinking about or be secretly worried about. It is included here as nothing more than an option to consider or to leave depending on your situation and views.

If we begin with the Islamic position on this topic. In terms of permissibility, polygyny is *allowed* in Islam: '...Then marry those that please you of [other] women, two or three or four. But if you fear that you will not be just, then [marry only] one or those your right hand possesses. That is more suitable that you may not incline [to injustice]' (Quran: 4:3). For many Muslims and non-Muslims, the issue of polygyny where a man has more than one wife is a contentious topic, but it's something Islam has *allowed* with clear guidelines for those that may want to consider it. The topic has many dimensions to be discussed depending on the circumstances of this permission and how this verse and historical practice should be interpreted today. Perhaps each case may require considering personal, social, and legal aspects accordingly, which are beyond the scope of this book.

Polygyny as an option concerning infertility has many factors to examine. I will share some of these factors below but there are bound to be others not mentioned as well.

Firstly, there is the ignorant belief, among many Muslim as well as non-Muslim communities, that infertility is always due to the female. This is not the reality, as shown in previous chapters, but the ignorant view of what infertility is and 'who to blame' means that many Muslims think a 'second wife' will fix the problem.

They think it will mean that the husband will automatically have biological children, but this isn't true, especially if the health issue is caused by a male factor. This misconception could lead a man to marry many women throughout his lifetime without ever being able to conceive a biological child.

Furthermore, many couples fall into the 'unexplained' category, which means there's no clear diagnosis for why pregnancy is not possible. Again, this means the husband marrying another woman doesn't guarantee he will have biological children since there's no known medical reason why he was unable to have children with the original wife.

Polygyny is an option for couples when the infertility is clearly caused by a female factor, but like all other options, there are several pros and cons to it.

One pro is that it allows the husband to essentially 'experiment' to see if he can have biological children with someone else. For a Muslim man desperate to have a child and keep his current household, this is a viable option that may bring a sense of hope to those involved.

Following on from that point, another pro is that a woman who is unable to conceive can find relief knowing her marriage can be maintained.

On the other side, a major con is the difficulty in navigating this for all those involved and who desire to be just.

If we first look at the possible hardships for the first wife to overcome in this situation, there's the possibility of feeling second best or being 'left' behind. It can't be easy for a woman who loves her husband and wants to have a family with him to watch him have that with someone else. Unfortunately, remarks and attitudes of family and the larger community may make it even worse for her.

Furthermore, some women feel blindsided and don't agree or wish to pursue this option but feel unable to express their feelings on the matter due to either pressure from the husband, family or society. She may also have some misplaced guilt on the issue of infertility and therefore feels trapped in the idea that this is her only option. For you my dear sister, the message is the same here as it is throughout this whole book: You must know and love yourself enough to protect your wishes and desires throughout every step of TTC experience. If you are in this situation, chapters 2, 8 and the section on guilt free life in chapter 6 are vital readings for you.

If we turn our attention to the husband now, he too is placed in an enormous struggle and possible heartache in this scenario. He may feel guilty and overwhelmed, worried that he has betrayed his wife by leaving her without a child whilst he goes on to start a family. He may also worry that she will think he rejected her, and for a man who loves his wife and wants to have a family with her, to deal with this emotionally is a hard toll.

Countless men choose to have multiple wives and children, but for a man who isn't necessarily choosing this, but rather feels compelled because of the situation, there is an enormous pressure financially and socially. For example, he must work through providing for two possible households which isn't easy for all men in this situation. This, coupled with now having to navigate being with two wives and potentially their families, is a huge job for men who want to be just and sincere.

Furthermore, some men worry about 'using' the second wife just to have a family, even if he plans on being good to her. The need for her as a 'necessity' rather than a choice can make it complicated.

Finally, let's turn our attention to the position of the second wife, who has been sought due to the necessity for children. It's easy to anticipate that she may feel some negativity about the situation.

It's quite clear that dealing with all these diverse issues and feelings for all involved is a difficult journey for a couple exploring this option.

It is also why those not in the marriage need to exercise extra sensitivity and caution in suggesting this option. However sincere advice and support can be very useful for some couples if, and when, they consider it.

Legally speaking, multiple spouses are against the law in the United Kingdom and many countries across the world. This means that only one wife is legally recognised by the state. However, for most Muslims, a *Nikah* completed in the Islamic tradition is sufficient to be married Islamically.

Numerous Muslim couples living in the UK and elsewhere don't register as legally married in their country of residence even when polygyny is not an issue. But let me be crystal clear here: under no circumstance can a man try to legally marry more than one wife at the same time, or he may be criminally investigated.

The legal position of the marriage in a scenario like polygyny is something that the potential wives need to investigate to determine safety and suitability for them and their lives.

Option 5: Divorce

This is the final option that I am including as a possible route to happiness or parenthood for a Muslim couple trying to conceive.

Not one option in this part of the book is designed to be easy. But by facing challenges head-on, centring ourselves deeply in understanding what we need and want as well as having on-going communication with our spouse, can we analyse and assess the suitability of each option.

There is a need to 'drown out' outside noise and place less importance on what you 'should' be doing, what is considered 'respectful', etc., and instead focus on what's best for you and your spouse.

My almost fanatic emphasis on the needs and wants for you and your spouse doesn't mean that you can't care about or have empathy for the sadness and loss that those around also feel. For sure, there are family and friends who desperately want the dream for you and hurt on your behalf. But in the end, the only feelings and opinions that should count in this scenario are the couple who are struggling to conceive.

We don't have to go through a divorce to appreciate how painful it can be. It's widely accepted that divorce is amongst the most stressful life events. University Hospital online listed it among their following top 5 stressful things:

- Death of a loved one
- Divorce
- Moving

- Major illness or injury
- Job loss

Despite all that, we still need to be brave enough to acknowledge this possibility if it is suitable for our circumstance. I'm sure you have heard about couples staying together for 8, 10, 15 years with no joy of children, then they separate, and at least one of them (if not both) go on to have biological children.

For example, there are two lovely souls within my circle that were married and tried to conceive for approximately 15 years. In the end, and with genuine heartbreak, they amicably and lovingly decided to divorce because they had no known medical reason not to conceive and both wanted to see what was possible.

It's over a decade later, and both have remarried and gone on to have biological children with their new spouses.

I don't for a minute doubt the amount of pain in their decision at the time, but the way things have unfolded means that they both received what they so desperately longed for.

The emotional chaos of having to divorce someone you love— someone whom you would have never contemplated divorce from were it not for the pressure of infertility—is heart-breaking. There may be a sense of 'giving up' that a couple in such a situation may have to work through as well. To have to move on and start again is excruciating to think about. However, humans are resilient, and, as in the above example, we have a way of getting used to change.

We must have faith in new opportunities and blessings which might be on the other side of divorce and beyond what we can imagine now.

I must stress, I am not encouraging divorce to anyone, especially not because of infertility.

However, despite the hardships that accompany even a civil divorce, we must recognise that it can be a positive step for some couples. As with all the options presented in this section, each couple must decide for themselves which option, if any, is suitable for them.

The option of divorce is impossible to contemplate for some but a reality for others. I have spoken with numerous women struggling with infertility who have either considered, are considering, or have gone through a divorce caused or cemented by the presence of infertility.

Just this week, I had conversation with an amazing woman who has just had her divorce finalised after 8 years of marriage and trying to conceive.

Naturally, it broke my heart to hear this. My heart broke for her and her now ex-husband. However, I saw it from a different perspective once I took the time to speak with her. I learnt that for her and her ex-husband there was a sense of freedom, a sense of healing, a sense of renewed possibilities for them. It felt like they were done with going round in circles and the pain of not conceiving as well as other misunderstandings. She was grateful for the availability of divorce. To start again. To trust the process that is life. To see what else is possible. Within her, I saw hope and I saw gratitude.

If you are contemplating this option or have gone through it, I pray for you to have strength and peace and a better outcome after it.

You may find comfort in the words of your Lord where the explanation and permissibility of divorce are followed with the following verses when he says: 'And will provide for him from where he does not expect. And whoever relies upon Allah - then He is sufficient for him. Indeed, Allah will accomplish His purpose. Allah has already set for everything a [decreed] extent' (Quran: 65:3).

***

EPILOGUE

A lot of food for thought has been given throughout this book. The ideas and possibilities recommended and provided are now yours to do with what you wish. Use the following questions to summarise for yourself your biggest take-aways from this book and some actions you will take moving forward.

1. What is one or more things that you have discovered from chapters 1-10 to use as tools to cope with infertility? This can include a mindset shift and challenging your thoughts.

2. What other blessings and opportunities exist in your life and how can you see or use them differently?

3. What is your overall goal in life right now and for the future apart from a baby? (e.g., happiness or self-acceptance or to fulfil your God-given purpose)

4. What do you need to do to achieve that goal? (e.g., what can give you happiness right now whilst still TTC?)

ENDNOTE

M any people wait to discuss major life struggles until they are on the other side of them. They want to share their stories with others that may be experiencing a similar struggle, but only from a place of safety. I get it.

They also want to wait until a 'good' outcome has been achieved (in this case healthy babies), so they can inspire hope for others, that their turn will arrive soon. They want to inspire them on what is possible and what is coming, and also 'how' to cope during the trial, but from the other side.

I understand the need for this approach. To be honest, I think that is why it has taken me over 10 years to write this book. I too was waiting to get to a place of safety where I could look back and share my wisdom on how to cope with infertility whilst you are in the thick of it.

I was struggling to see the benefit of sharing my story, of sharing any tools of support, before I had my own 'happy ending'. I was also scared. I was scared for my emotional well-being. To delve deep into this book and all the parts of trying to conceive have not been easy. I was worried I was not strong enough, but this is exactly why it had to happen this way, at this time.

I wanted to share this book with you whilst I was in the thick of the struggle with you. I realised there is a great benefit to gaining insight as well as hope from those still in your shoes. From those who are surviving it, whilst you are also trying to survive it.

I think there is hope here too. On the journey itself. I don't want to pause happiness, hope, or joy until 'then'. I don't want to pause providing support and receiving it until 'then'. I want to remind myself and fiercely encourage you to find and fight for joy now. For support now. For hope now, whilst we continue this journey together.

I am not speaking to you in hindsight and rationally advising you on how best to cope with this hardship. That would be too easy. I am in the fight with you and I think the power and the need lie here.